CW01023412

DIGITAL EPIDEMIOLOGY

AN INTRODUCTION TO DISEASE SURVEILLANCE USING DIGITAL DATA

Mark D. Walker

Sicklebrook Publishing, Sheffield, U.K.

ISBN: 978-1-4709-2036-4

CONTENTS

DEDICATION

I would like to dedicate this work to my father, David Harry Walker, who my family lost early in 2022. I began writing this book in the period after our loss. It is for him.

ABOUT THE AUTHOR

I am a zoologist based in Sheffield, U.K. I have worked on a wide range of field research projects, mostly studying parasites and their hosts. This led inevitably to me becoming interested in parasitic disease, and from that to infectious disease more generally. I was exited by the new and novel sources of data that could be used to learn about disease, and thus became interested in digital epidemiology. I have published a variety of research, some using the sources and methods described in this book. Much of this research is related to COVID-19 or the influence the pandemic has had on other conditions.

PREFACE

After becoming interested in how internet search data could be used to study disease, I sought out a short introductory text on the topic. I wanted a brief description of the new digital tools and methods that were being used to understand where disease occurs and among whom. But I could find none. There were many research papers using the methods I was interested in, but I could find no single text which tried to synthesize this information in one text. So I have tried to write one myself!

A major problem was deciding what to include and what to leave out. I quickly realized that a comprehensive text was impossible. The sheer weight of publications and research being conducted meant that this was simply not feasible. I aimed to write no more than 100 pages, with around 100 key references. I have failed. However, I have hopefully still managed to provide an overview that remains short and concise, but one which still provides an impression of what digital epidemiology is, what it entails, and where it is going.

The emphasis is on disease surveillance: can disease outbreaks be spotted using novel digital resources? Can trends in disease occurrence be identified using such data?

The book aims to:

- Provide an overview: The first chapter is a general introduction to digital epidemiology, defining what it is and why it developed. A number of authors have written on digital epidemiology, and this is my interpretation of their work.

- Data sources, important methods: The following chapters detail new data sources and some of the methods used to interpret them.

- Key references: I aim to provide a selection of references, rather than a complete literature review for each topic. I try to provide a mix of notable early studies, and others that are interesting or more recent. Following prevailing trends I provide a minimum of reviews.

I have tried to provide as wide a range of examples from as many countries as possible, but please be aware I am based in the U.K. and this may affect my choices.

I produced this text with no external or institutional support, so please have understanding of its limitations. I had no one to ask for help. It is difficult to produce such a text independently. I have tried the best I can.

Each chapter should be considered more an essay providing a light introduction to the topic rather than an academic text. My target audience is someone wishing to learn more about this field and this text should be used as a basis for further study. Please use it to start more in depth research of your own. I hope it provokes thought and comment. Please send me constructive ideas and comments for improvement.

Mark Walker, Sheffield, U.K.
mark_david_walker@yahoo.co.uk

1

WHAT IS DIGITAL EPIDEMIOLOGY?

...there is one area where the world isn't making much progress: pandemic preparedness.

Bill Gates, 2018.

Epidemiology is the science of disease; how it is distributed, how many people are affected by it, and what the underlying causes of it are (BMJ, 2022). Essentially, epidemiology looks at how often disease occurs in defined groups or populations of people, examines how this compares to other groups, then tries to look for the reasons for any differences. Such knowledge is important in preventing disease and illness. It is also essential in helping control or limit the spread of disease if it is infectious in nature. Such epidemiological knowledge can be used to guide healthcare provision and management.

This has always been a broad discipline attracting people with diverse skill sets and of different scientific backgrounds. Maybe the classic stereotype of a disease scientist is of a microbiologist working in a laboratory studying viral pathogens down a microscope. However, epidemiology can also involve a wide range of specialists from a wide variety of disciplines. Entomologists study the lifecycle of mosquitoes in remote parts of Africa. Skilled mathematicians also often play a role in epidemiology, meticulously maintaining records on reported cases and using statistical techniques to understand patterns and trends in disease occurrence. Sociologists can be involved in epidemiology, studying people's habits and lifestyles in order to understand why certain groups of people are at greater risk of certain diseases and not others.

What does epidemiology do?:
- Outbreak detection: identification of where disease outbreaks begin.
- Public health surveillance: ascertaining the prevalence of disease among a population.
- Investigation: study of the underlying reasons for differences in disease occurrence.

WHAT IS 'DIGITAL EPIDEMIOLOGY'?
This book introduces the emerging field of digital epidemiology. Our entire lives have been revolutionized by technological developments over the last 30 years. These include the development of personal computing, the now almost ubiquitous use of the internet, and the widespread uptake of the mobile phone. These technologies have changed how we work, how we live and crucially, how we think about the world. We can now all be said to be living in a digital age.

The study of disease has similarly been affected by these technological changes. Today efforts to understand the diseases which affect us are as likely to be done behind a computer screen as in a microbiology laboratory or clinic. The basis of digital epidemiology is, as the name implies, digital data. Epidemiology has always been heavily underpinned by data and statistics. However, the data used to study disease today is now rarely kept on paper. It is mostly held digitally, often remotely, and is easily shareable at the click of a button around the globe. We are living in the age of big data, machine learning and artificial intelligence.

Many of these technological developments have simply extended what traditional epidemiology does; for example epidemiologists have always been interested in weather and climate and how this affects rates of certain conditions. But the advent of digital records means the scope of such study is far wider than before. There are now more detailed records, on more parameters, over longer periods of time. Digital epidemiology has broadened both the scope of what information can be used to understand health, where it can be obtained from, and who can be involved.

But some technological developments have opened up major and interesting new avenues, which have greatly extended the scope of traditional epidemiological research. A wide range of new information and data sources, on topics never previously considered of much interest in the study of disease, are now available. There has been a gradual realization that information, often not directly related to epidemiology at all, can be used to learn more about disease. For example can people's shopping habits tell us about the illnesses they will experience in the future? Can we predict epidemics on the basis of internet searching? Can we estimate how fast a disease will spread into a new city based on data on the number of bus journeys made in a country? Such information and data was not previously considered relevant to epidemiology.

As mentioned above, epidemiologists come from a range of disciplines. Here we concentrate on a new type of professional that has entered the epidemiological arena; the data scientist. We examine how this new professional is contributing to epidemiology today. The management and understanding of data has developed greatly in recent decades, in tandem with developments in computing in general. Only 20 years ago there was little awareness of what data science was. Yet in 2012 being a data scientist was considered one of the 'sexiest' careers there was (Davenport and Patil, 2012).

Essentially, digital epidemiology has the same objectives as traditional epidemiology; to better understand the reasons why disease occurs where it does and among whom it does. Where does disease occur? Who has or is at risk of a particular disease? Where do they live? How can this best be ascertained and studied, recorded and mapped? What is different is the method and manner of working.

Epidemiology examines both communicable disease, those that can be transmitted from person to person, and non communicable diseases, those conditions that develop typically due to lifestyle. In this text the emphasis is on communicable diseases and in particular disease surveillance and outbreak detection. Many of the new methods have proved particularly useful for investigating those conditions that spread from person to person and understanding when outbreaks occur. These include some of the most challenging conditions that affect humankind; perhaps the most obvious of which is malaria. The World Health Organization estimated that in 2020 there were 241 million malaria cases worldwide, leading to an estimated 627,000 deaths (WHO, 2021). Such figures should make those living in the 'developed West' feel uncomfortable, at the very least.

DEFINING DIGITAL EPIDEMIOLOGY

It helps if we start by defining what digital epidemiology is. This subject area was not conceived or invented; it simply evolved as a new discipline as new data sources became available and technological improvements meant new ways of obtaining and using data became available. Who first identified that epidemiology was changing in this way?

As the internet grew in scope and size it was quickly realized that this offered new opportunities for those studying disease. Eysenach (2002) conceived the name 'infodemiology', abbreviated from 'information epidemiology' to describe these new sources of data:

> Infodemiology can be defined as the science of distribution and determinants of information in an electronic medium, specifically the internet, or in a population, with the ultimate aim to inform public health and public policy.

However, this is somewhat narrow in scope and was conceived principally with internet search data in mind. Who could have predicted how the range and scope of digital data sources would grow further? Although much of the information used in digital epidemiology is later made available on the internet, often it originates from non-internet based sources. For example, think of mobile phone tracking records, which are collected by communications companies, but which are not typically available on the internet.

A good date for the start of digital epidemiology was a paper resulting from a workshop on data science and epidemiology organized at Penn State University in 2011 (Salanthé et al. 2012). This used the name digital epidemiology and outlined some key developments that were changing disease science; notably the continued development of the internet, the mobile phone, and data mining. Salanthé (2018) provided a broader definition of what digital epidemiology was, and attempted to encompass the plethora of information sources becoming available, not only those accessible through the internet:

> Digital epidemiology is epidemiology that uses data that was generated outside the public health system, i.e. with data that was not generated with the primary purpose of doing epidemiology.

These articles led to an increase in awareness of digital epidemiology. However, this definition remains limited in that today many public health professionals are actively generating the data they use in their research with epidemiology in mind. The data they are collecting is no afterthought of a non-epidemiologist.

In a commentary article Eckhof and Tatem (2015) took a broader view as to what it constitutes:

> Digital epidemiology can be broadly defined as epidemiology that uses digital methods from data collection to data analysis.

Velasco (2018) also emphasized the digital aspect, but concentrated only on disease surveillance, defining digital epidemiology as:

> the use of digital means for the purposes of – and the monitoring, research, analysis, and decision making implicit in – disease surveillance.

Here is an alternative:

> Digital epidemiology involves answering questions about population level disease and health, using remotely or automatically collected sources of data, which are in a digitized format.

We all know what it is like to feel ill. However, today we have the ability to tell the entire world about it. We can post about our feelings online, search for symptoms and treatments, read about the experiences of others who have similar conditions, then order medicine, and book a doctors appointment online. Doing all these things leaves an electronic trail of evidence behind us which can be used to study patterns in disease and health. These are the ingredients of digital epidemiology.

SIMILAR TOPICS, ALTERNATIVE NAMES: Digital health, eHealth, mHealth

In recognition that health science was changing, the World Health Organization issued its first guidelines relating to the use of digital technology for health in 2019 (WHO, 2019). These guidelines examined some of the names used to denote digital methods of working. Various names have developed depending on the technology being used and the specific areas being examined. The popularity of these has varied. Other names that have gained popularity when referring to technology and healthcare include 'eHealth', 'digital health' and 'mHealth'.

'eHealth' is often used to denote improvements to individual healthcare that have occurred through technological and digital developments. WHO (2019) defines eHealth broadly as:

> the use of information and communications technology in support of health and health-related fields.

However, despite this broad description, eHealth is generally often used only to refer to internet based aspects of healthcare. This name does not seem to have caught the imagination to the same extent as others and appears to be falling out of favour.

'mHealth' refers to healthcare based around mobile phone, or smartphone, technology. The 'm' referring to 'Mobile'. WHO (2019) define mHealth simply as:

> the use of mobile wireless technologies for health.

Another name, 'digital health', is now also well established. It can be defined as the various ways technological progress improves healthcare. The scope of digital health is thus large and can encompass everything from the development of health related internet sites, health apps allowing personal monitoring of health, as well as health related 'wearables' such as the FitBit (Velesco, 2018). Generally the name digital health is used to encompass all ways in which technological progress help healthcare, and often includes both eHealth and mHealth.

In comparison digital epidemiology can be differentiated from these other terms by being considered as the use of technology for the study of disease at a population level, rather than aiding individual care and treatment. It is principally involved with disease surveillance, quantification of disease occurrence, and comparison at the population level. Arguably, there is much overlap between digital health, mHealth and digital epidemiology. For example, improved disease diagnosis through smartphone technology obviously helps individual healthcare, but could also conceivably improve disease surveillance by allowing quicker notification of public health officials.

Arguably, education and communication about health and disease are topics important in both epidemiology and to healthcare providers. Tools such as the internet can play a large part in encouraging education and thus combating disease. It is therefore important to consider the wider implications of technological developments, and all the ways in which they can aid health.

THE FOUNDATIONS OF DIGITAL EPIDEMIOLOGY

Unlike some disciplines whose conception can be traced back to a single discovery or sole inspired researcher, no single invention or development can be seen as marking the start of digital epidemiology. It has evolved as a discipline due to a multitude of developments, each of which have played a part in improving disease science. One can argue about which development was the most important, but they all played in part in its formation. Key developments on the road to digital epidemiology include:

Personal computing

The invention of the microprocessor is often cited as allowing the beginning of personal computing. Its invention is often attributed to Ted Hoff and a team of researchers at Intel. The microprocessor first came onto the market in 1971. Its invention meant that the mass production of small personal computers was possible. Before this time computers were expensive and large machines. Those made in the 1940's and 1950's could take up entire rooms and weighed several tons.

However, the widespread use of personal computers for work purposes only really began from the early 1990's. Key in its development was the work of Microsoft, founded in 1975 by Bill Gates and Paul Allen. The company concentrated on the development of operating systems, with MS-DOS from 1980, which later became the Windows operating system. The release of Windows 95 is a good candidate milestone for the start of mass personal computing. Also important was the work of Apple. The Mackintosh Classic, developed by Apple, was available from 1990 and had a retail price of less than $1,000.

Digitization

Over much of historical time records have been kept on paper. Although fairly permanent and long lasting there are obvious disadvantages. Obviously if there is only a single 'hard' copy, the number of people able to access it is limited. Communication of such information is limited. The growing availability of personal computers meant that a new way of record keeping began to exist.

Today records are increasingly being held on electronic databases with no hard copy being kept at all. This improves accuracy, makes life easier for those managing such data, and increases accessibility. It is easier to move data between people, and to make multiple copies. Data is now more widely available and more easy to manipulate than ever before.

Social media

From the 2000's it became possible to communicate easily with a person living thousands of miles away and discuss such topics as our hopes, fears, and ideas, to explore different cultures and share ideas. Instead most people seem to send each other images of meals or funny pictures of dogs on surfboards! If nothing else social media shows that humans are innately social. Social media sites offer a social medium, online.

The main characteristic of social media is that it contains user generated content. For the first time rather than being a consumer of information, a person can be a creator. Social media encompasses blogs, image and video sharing services (YouTube), gaming sites and collaborative work projects (Wikipedia). However, when most people think of social media they think immediately of social networking sites (Facebook, Twitter). The development of each of these is described in subsequent chapters.

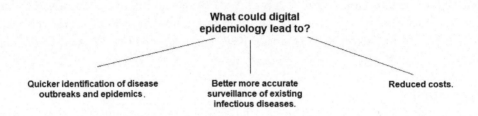

Mobile phones

The first commercially available phone was the Motorola DynaTAC 8000X which appeared in 1973. This resembled a brick. Martin Cooper working for the technology company Motorola is often cited as the inventor of the mobile phone which occurred in the early 1970's. However, the development of mobile communication had a much longer history, mainly being driven forward by the military from the 1940's who required improved communication for forces in field combat situations.

From the digital epidemiology viewpoint it is the 'smartphone' that is proving most interesting. Smartphones contain some computing capacity, principally allowing the ability to access the internet. They may also contain cameras able to take high quality photographs. The Nokia 9000 communicator which became available from 1996 and the Ericsson R380, which was available from 2000, heralded the start of modern mass and on-the-go internet access. These developments meant that from being an oddity and the preserve of businessmen in the early 2000, mobile and smartphone ownership is now pretty much ubiquitous.

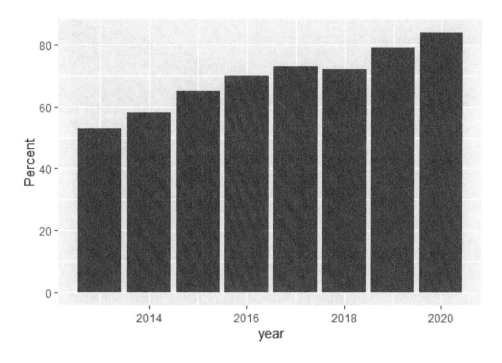

Smartphone possession: the percentage of the Great British population accessing the internet 'on-the-go' using a smartphone (2013 to 2019), or using a smartphone for private use (2020). Data from the Office for National Statistics, U.K. Internet access: households and individuals, annual reports (2020).

The internet and world wide web

The internet has its roots in a military communications network, which enabled communication between remote computers. Its beginnings stem from the late 1960's when Massachusetts Institute of Technology (MIT) researchers along with those from the U.S. Department of Defence Advanced Research Projects Agency established a global computer network known as ARPANET. This began in 1969. However, before a truly international net could be created what was needed were global standards and methods of linking computers together. Throughout the 1970's protocols for such linkage were developed and a method of sending data using UNIX was standardized. In 1983 the Transfer Control Protocol/Internetwork Protocol was adopted by ARPANET, and this date is often cited as the start of the internet as we know it today. Local Area Networks were developed in the 1980's which made the system resilient because it was based on multiple regional networks.

The world wide web itself stems from the European Organization for Nuclear Research (CERN) where Tim Berners-Lee helped developed Hyper Text Markup Language (HTML) and Uniform Resource Locator (URL) in the 1980's. 1995 was to prove a pivotal year for the nascent web as Windows 95 was launched, which heralded the era of personal computing. The language Java, which enabled interesting websites that contained animation, also became available in this year.

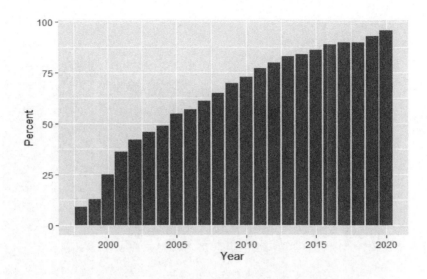

**Households with internet access in Great Britain
(Office for National Statistics, 2020).**

Data science

One definition of data science from the IBM Cloud Education team is that it is:

> a multidisciplinary approach to extracting actionable insights from the large and ever-in creasing volumes of data.

Basically data science is the scientific study of data; it consists of the extraction, collation, formatting, then analysis of data. Data science is based upon the skills and knowledge from a variety of scientific disciplines including mathematics, statistics, and computing. Domain specific knowledge is also important in knowing exactly what data is useful and what it is showing in each specific context. Awareness that data science was a distinct and recognizable discipline in its own right developed from the early 2000's.

Statistics has always been the bedrock of infectious disease epidemiology. The developments in digital technology meant that traditional data sources could be improved, or combined with others, to improve the standards and eliminate shortcomings present in traditional datasets.

'Big data'

Increases in computing power led to the ability to collect, handle and store previously unimaginable amounts of data. Consider the storage capacity of the principal methods of saving data over the last 50 years, and how the amount of data that can be saved has increased over time:

1986	IBM floppy disc	720 KB
2011	San Disc Cruzer	4 gb
2022	Cloud computing	Practically unlimited

14

A widely used definition of big data from IBM (2022) is that it is:

> data whose scale, diversity, and complexity require new architecture, techniques, algorithms, and analytics to manage it and extract value and hidden knowledge from it

Another widely used definition from Andreu-Perez (2015) is that big data is a:

> massive amount of structured and unstructured data

So basically 'big data' could be considered simply as large volumes of data? Actually it is more than just this. 'Big data' is often characterized by the four V's: volume, velocity, variety, and veracity:

- Volume: as the name suggests, there is a lot of it! Just imagine how many emails are sent each day. Imagine a sensor recording weather temperatures instantaneously every minute; before long you have a large dataset. How many mobile phones calls are made each day?

- Variety: data comes from everywhere. Data is now not just numbers. Think of photos, images, and sounds.

- Velocity: refers to the speed at which data can be downloaded or streamed.

- Veracity: previously data was collected for specific research purposes. Big data is collected because it is there. Why? Maybe it will be useful for something.....

In the medical realm, big data can come from a variety of sources. Lee and Yoon (2017) list just some, including administrative claim records, clinical registries, electronic health records, bio-metric data, patient-reported data, the internet, medical imaging, biomarker data, prospective cohort studies, and large clinical trials. Obviously the availability of all this data opens up new research possibilities. However, just as important as a datasets size, is the possibility of it interacting in previously unimagined ways with other datasets, thus leading to new discoveries and findings (Lee and Yoon, 2017).

But there are potential problems and disadvantages with big data. Traditionally research data was carefully managed. It was difficult, expensive and time consuming to obtain high quality research data. Thus, data collection was specific and targeted, with great care being taken to ensure it was done correctly. But much big data is collected simply because it is there and because it can be collected with little effort. It is collected simply as a by-product. It could well not show what is required, or what one thinks. Quantity does not equate to quality.

Data 'mining'
As explained above, instead of being data collectors, scientists are becoming more data curators. More important than the collection, is deciding what is important to keep, what to examine, and deciding which data to use to answer specific research questions.

Data mining is a term used to denote the analysis of databases to extract data of interest and discovering patterns from it (IBM, 2022). Iavindrasana et al. (2009) lists a number of steps in the data mining process. These include dataset selection, preparing data for examination through 'data cleaning', deciding what to do with outliers, and choosing important variables. Some of these steps have become highly specialized, using methods such as bootstrapping and cross validation to systematically examine portions of a dataset in a systematic manner. Machine learning and deep learning techniques can be used to organize and filter data.

Data accessibility and management

Traditionally data was guarded most carefully, almost secretively, by scientists. Data used to cost a lot of time and money to obtain and was therefore a valuable resource. Even fragments of data could yield important findings and result in important publications.

Today, because data is everywhere the rules have changed. Because now the problem is being able to identify what is useful and the best ways to work with what you have, collaboration is now more important than guarding data. Maybe someone can interpret the data better than you? So the sharing of data has become commonplace, and facilities such as GitHub, which allows the storage and sharing of data have promoted this.

Algorithms, machine learning and artificial intelligence

An algorithm is nothing complicated or novel. It is merely a list of steps or instructions required in order to complete some specific task or solve a problem. Algorithms have a long history, being used by both the Babylonians and Ancient Greeks. The Persian mathematician Abu Abdullah Muhammad ibn Musa Al-Khwarizmi is credited with their naming. In the modern era Alan Turing is credited with highlighting their importance in the realm of computing.

Algorithms are an important part of machine learning. This is basically asking the computer to make forecasts and predictions based on the data you give it. However, the user decides which algorithms the computer should use to solve them.

Geographic Information Systems

Another important development for epidemiology were Geographic Information Systems, routinely simply referred to as GIS. These are specialized programs which allow the visualization and analysis of spatial data. In essence, they allow the creation of maps, with the user being able to add layers and features as desired.

GIS software which allowed users of personal computers to develop maps began to be developed in the 1970's, but only became widely available in the 1990's. Popular programs include the Windows based ArcGis, QGIS, and the open source GRASS software. Together with the wider availability of environmental data, such as that through remote sensing, it has been possible to map areas of likely disease incidence.

KEY DEVELOPMENTS IN THE EARLY HISTORY OF DIGITAL EPIDEMIOLOGY

It is difficult to track the early development of digital epidemiology. In many cases, new technology was used simply to enhance traditional research. Who was the first researcher to use spreadsheets to manage records of disease occurrence? In many cases the methods used were not new, but simply new computing capability meant that these techniques could be implemented much easier than before. Additionally, tracing the beginning of digital epidemiology is difficult because it covers so many potential techniques and methods. It is difficult to determine how the use of each developed. Here as some of the main milestones in the progression of digital epidemiology.

Before 2000

Program for Monitoring Emerging Diseases: ProMed mail

Many authors cite the development of ProMed mail in 1994 as the start of the digital epidemiological age. The Program for Monitoring Emerging Diseases, known simply as ProMed mail, is an email based news and reporting system which aims to connect epidemiologists across the globe. It helps raise awareness of disease outbreaks, providing an early warning system for problems with a potentially wider impact. Once signed up, users receive regular email alerts which detail disease outbreaks across the globe.

Global Public Health Intelligence Network: GPHIN

Another early example of digital epidemiology is the Global Public Health Intelligence Network (GPHIN), established in 1997. GPHIN was developed by the Canadian Public Health authorities, as there contribution to the World Health Organization disease surveillance efforts. It is an informal news network, providing email alerts of potential disease outbreaks and health problems worldwide. Information is gathered from websites, social media and online news forums, with news of disease outbreaks being relayed as informal reports between a network of epidemiologists. Rather unfortunately resources appear to have been diverted away from GPHIN in the Spring of 2019, which meant it failed to provide alerts relating to COVID-19. But from late 2020 resources were again reallocated and alerts began being issued again.

Both ProMed mail and GPHIN proved useful in helping track the Severe Acute Respiratory Syndrome 'SARS' outbreak which started late in 2002 in south east China. This helped both inform scientists and public health officials globally about this problem, thus helping in the response to the outbreak (Brownstein et al. 2009).

The Global Outbreak Alert and Response Network: GOARN

The World Health Organization established the Global Outbreak Alert and Response Network (GOARN) in April 2000 at a meeting in Geneva in an attempt to improve the international response to disease outbreaks. The idea was to establish a common framework for action when outbreaks occurred, improve communication about outbreaks between countries, and facilitate sharing of technical and expert knowledge. GOARN almost immediately proved useful in the SARS outbreak of 2002 and 2003, and later in Africa following the Ebola outbreaks in 2014. GOARN is an excellent example of how improved communication has improved disease surveillance and the public health response to outbreaks.

2000 to 2010

Bio-terrorism and syndromic surveillance

Did terrorism provide a key impetus to the development of digital epidemiology? Following the 2001 September 11 terrorist attacks in the U.S. the fear of terrorism was in the forefront of many people's minds. In addition to the September attacks, a series of anthrax attacks also occurred during 2001 in the U.S. An unknown individual posted letters containing anthrax spores through the U.S. postal system resulting in several deaths. Although relatively small scale, the potential for a much larger attack was evident. What if someone repeated such a bio-terrorist attack, but across a wider area or affected a far larger number of people? How could this be quickly identified and the focal point found?

Identifying and tracing individuals affected in the anthrax attacks was difficult. Conventional methods of spotting disease could easily miss outbreaks of such rarely occurring conditions. Medical doctors, for example, could easily overlook cases of anthrax, as it is not something they see routinely. Instead it was realized that there was a need to use non-orthodox methods instead.

Thus, there was an increase in interest in syndromic surveillance. Syndromic surveillance can be defined as the study of the occurrence of symptoms potentially indicative of a specific illness (Henning, 2004). This helps spot potential illness clusters before they are reported through official channels. It also allows effective control and treatment to be initiated as early as possible, thus containing disease transmission and mitigating its effects. The underlying principle is that symptoms begin to appear before someone seeks out medical advice and a diagnosis is made. Development of syndromic surveillance systems thus requires knowledge of the suite of symptoms associated with specific conditions.

Whether bio-terrorism was an important factor initiating development of digital epidemiology techniques or not, the potential to combat terrorism at least provided a good justification to obtain funding for early research studies. If nothing else, these early studies on syndromic surveillance emphasized that the epidemiological landscape was changing and new methods of working were becoming available.

Health Map

Quickly understanding information which is in a text format can take time. Visualizing data makes interpreting data much easier, either through the use of graphs, pictures, or maps. Health Map was started in September 2006, and mapped known incidents of disease thus making it easier to understand where disease outbreaks were occurring and possibly spot clusters or other related patterns (Brownstein et al 2008).

This resource collates data from official sources, such as the European Centre for Disease Control, then simply maps where they occur. It provides users with information on outbreaks listed to near to where they have been in the recent past. It also integrates news and media reports on disease outbreaks. HealthMap quickly became well known among epidemiologists.

Google Flu Trends

Influenza, known informally as 'flu', is a most problematic infectious condition in that the impact it has can vary considerably each year. In the young it is often a relatively mild illness. But in the old and vulnerable it can be much more serious, leading to a range of complications and often resulting in death. As if it was not bad enough that influenza causes a significant number of deaths each year, equally as serious can be the knock-on effects seen in bad years. The large numbers suffering influenza who require treatment can block up medical facilities, filling beds and wards to capacity and beyond. Medical staff then start to fall ill and be absent from work, only exacerbating problems. The side effects of an overwhelmed health care system can cause just as many deaths as the influenza does itself directly.

How bad will each seasons outbreak be? Can this be predicted? Being able to forecast whether the influenza burden in a given year will be severe or not, and in which specific locations it will peak and when, could mean resources are more effectively allocated leading to the saving of thousands of lives.

Originally conceived as a tool to aid marketing, Google Trends (beginning as Google Trends for Insight) provides the volume of internet searching on certain keywords for specific locations over time. In 2006, Roni Zeiger, a scientist working at Google, conceived Google Flu Trends to track influenza using search results for important search terms from Google Trends. This could help forecast when cases would peak and where. The methodology gained rapid notoriety (Ginsberg et a. 2009). However, questions about the accuracy of Google Flu Trends soon started to be raised; particularly after 2012 when it overestimated forecasted case numbers during the 2012 to 2013 influenza season. However, potentially just as important as the project itself was that it raised awareness about what was possible using new sources of data and new methods of statistical analysis.

Twitter and Facebook

Another leap forward for digital epidemiology was the development of social media platforms, of which Twitter and Facebook are two of the most well-known. These opened up a whole new avenue for researchers to investigate, including the study of personal feelings, wellness and whether users were well or not. An obvious challenge was dealing with the large volume of data such platforms generated.

2010 to 2020

The birth of digital epidemiology

By the end of the 2000's there was a growing awareness that new methods were opening up in epidemiology with a number of review and commentary articles commenting on the new developments that were occurring. Widely cited is the article by Brownstein et al. (2009). John Brownstein, a professor at Harvard Medical School and Boston Children's Hospital, is one of the leading lights in the field of digital epidemiology, and is cited as one of the first computational epidemiologists. The 2009 article summarized a number of the developing data sources, such as Blogs and Web searching, and identified that these new sources had to potential to supplement traditional epidemiology.

The decade between 2010 and 2020 signalled the birth of digital epidemiology in name as well as spirit. Already mentioned in this text, and widely cited as being the originator of the moniker 'digital epidemiology' was the scientist Marcel Salanthé. He even calls himself a 'digital epidemiologist'. In his early 'digital epidemiological' research he examined influenza and found that tweets and news reports mirrored case reports (Salanthé et al. 2013). However, others also highlighted the growing influence that digital technology was having on disease science as a discipline. For example, in a heavily cited review article Millonovich et al. (2014) noted the great increase in internet usage globally and the opportunities this presented to those interested in disease occurrence.

DELSI: Digital epidemiology; its ethical, legal and social implications
Notably, a symposium using the title 'digital epidemiology' took place in 2015 in Berlin. Organized by the German public health centre, the Robert Koch Institute, this aimed to bring together a small group of leading epidemiologists to study the ethics of using digital technology in disease surveillance. It concentrated on the ethical and social implications of the newly developing technologies, topics of particular importance in Germany due to its historical past. The articles published after this meeting are an important first port of call for those interested in digital epidemiology. In the symposium Eckmanns and Hempel (2015) asked:

> Does the use of emerging technologies and digital tools, especially big data, present an epistemic shift in epidemiology?

2020 to today

The COVID-19 revolution
War is often cited as being the catalyst for innovation. Can a disease pandemic be considered as having the same effect on epidemiological science? When the COVID-19 virus, officially named Coronavirus disease 2019, began to spread globally in late 2019, the entire scientific community worldwide was initiated into action. The potential threat even caused scientists and inventors not involved in disease science to divert their attention to finding ways to understand, control and treat this virus and the disease.

For example, following a a request for ventilators from the British Government, the British inventor and entrepreneur James Dyson, famous for inventing the bag less vacuum cleaner bearing his name, tasked his research team with developing a new type of machine. A large surge in COVID-19 patients was expected, and ventilators were needed in their care. The result was the invention of a new ventilator; the CoVent, developed in only 10 days (Liu et al. 2021).

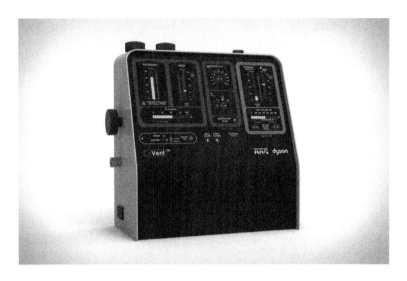

Rapid ingenuity in the face of crisis: The Dyson Covent ventilator, invented in response to the COVID-19 crisis.

In many cases the technologies implemented in response to COVID-19 simply used techniques that had been developed over the previous 20 years. It required only the emergence of a pandemic for these to demonstrate they had reached maturity. For example, use of mobile phone technology was key in the ZOE COVID Symptom Study developed in the U.K. and U.S., which allowed participants to submit details of potential symptoms. In the early days of the pandemic when the clinical course of infection in those progressing to serious disease was not known, such information was invaluable. This study identified loss of smell, anosmia, as being a symptom indicative of infection (Menni et al. 2020). This and other similar studies allowed the identification of potential infection hot spots and an estimation to be made as to the size of outbreaks.

Also notable during the pandemic was the development of 'contact tracing' systems. Previously this phrase was only understood and used by those with epidemiological training. But the pandemic led to it becoming used by the wider general public. Traditionally, contact tracing by epidemiologists was a manual process. Involving physically finding people, then urging them to remember people they had been in close proximity tob, who were then in turn contacted. Developments such as smartphones with Bluetooth technology, opened up the possibility of creating automated processes, with individuals being contacted automatically when someone they had been in close proximity to had tested positive. Throughout the pandemic a number of systems were developed in various nations worldwide. However, the question as to whether they were truly effective remains open (Braithwaite et al. 2020). Typically for such systems to be effective there needs to be a high uptake of users among the population.

The pandemic helped show how digitized the world had become. For example, between 2020 and 2022 there were more than 17 million visits every month to COVID-19 web pages of the British National Health Service (NHS)(Nuffield Trust, 2022). As of August 2022 there had been 1 billion visits to NHS websites by people seeking information on COVID-19.

Key epidemiological and technological developments.

Year	Epidemiological Development or Key Event	Technological development
1994	ProMed Mail	
1995		Windows 95 released. Yahoo! And Amazon begin. Java allows animated websites.
1996		
1997	GPHIN	
1998		
1999		
2000		
2001	Anthrax Bio-terrorist Attacks in U.S.A.	
2002	SARS outbreak in South East Asia	
2003		
2004		Mark Zuckerberg starts Facebook
2005		
2006	HealthMap Mumps epidemic	Twitter started March 2006 Google Trends launched.
2007		Fitbit founded 2007
2008	Google Flu Trends began	
2009	The Global Outbreak Alert and Response Network (GOARN) established. H1N1 virus 'Swine Flu' influenza pandemic	
2010		
2011	Pertussis epidemic begins.	
2012	Marcle Salanthé uses name 'Digital epidemiology' Middle East respiratory syndrome MERS outbreak in the Middle East	
2013	2013 to 2016 West African Ebola virus outbreak.	
2014		
2015	DELSI Digital Epidemiology symposium	
2016	Zika virus, notably in South America	
2017		
2018		
2019	The COVID-19 pandemic begins	
2020		

ADVANTAGES OF DIGITAL EPIDEMIOLOGY

Democratic epidemiology

Previously only those present at, or affiliated with, an academic or governmental institution could participate and contribute to epidemiological research. Access to the data, literature and knowledge required to learn about disease was restricted to those in such institutions. A good example is provided by academic journals, which in earlier times could only be accessed by reading the 'hard copy' at an academic library. The general public were to the greater degree excluded from such knowledge.

The internet and world wide web has meant such knowledge is now much more freely available. The old business models of scientific journals has been challenged, with scientific work being much easier to share and make freely available. Now, it is possible for anyone to download academic journal articles themselves, or even obtain the data needed for research.

This has greatly widened the range of people able to undertake such research. The online website Kaggle provides an excellent example of how science is becoming increasingly democratic. This website allows those with an interest in data science to share ideas, code and compete in coding competitions for fun and sometimes even cash! Topics related to disease diagnosis are a common theme in projects. Datasets related to various medical topics are regularly uploaded and made accessible for anyone to work with and study. These developments mean that people with different skills sets and ideas can contribute to research. This means new ideas can be generated and shared more easily.

Remote epidemiology

On a similar vein, previously in order to complete research on disease you typically needed to be close geographically to either an academic centre where knowledge was obtainable or close to the location where cases of disease were occurring. For example, if you wanted to study the factors affecting the distribution of the insect vectors of malaria, then you actually had to get out in the field and collect the data. For the most part this required (for European scientists) extended periods of fieldwork in foreign locations.

Digital epidemiology has changed this. Data can be collected remotely, automatically, and instantly, without a researcher needing to go to much physical effort to obtain it. Often now all that is needed is access to the internet, and off you go! A scientist based in Europe is able to study parasite vectors often without foreign travel (sadly). This has widened the pool of talent able to conduct research; remember most scientists are northern hemisphere based, yet many of the Neglected Tropical Diseases tend to be in the southern hemisphere.

Cost

Producing data through 'fieldwork' or through direct contact with patients, as is often the case in traditional epidemiology is expensive. To adequately monitor and control disease, professionals able to identify and record disease are required on the ground where it occurs. Think of a traditional sentinel surveillance system based on family medical practitioner surgeries. Behind these there needs to be a network of administrators, recording data, keeping records, and collating it for analysis on a national level. This is expensive.

Many of the data sources used in digital epidemiology are free to access. Think of data from Google Trends. Digital epidemiology can streamline the process of obtaining data, removing many of the people required on the path from data collection to data analysis, making it a much cheaper form of science.

Speed

Traditional epidemiology can be slow. Imagine a clinician spotting a potentially infectious condition in a patient they see. Even without any laboratory testing, it can still take time for information on this suspected case to pass through the official data recording processes, and reach local public health officials who can then initiate a response. Official notification takes time. In the U.K. weekly reports of notifiable diseases are produced, however in the case of infectious diseases even a week can be enough time for outbreaks to become well established. If you add to this the complications and delays inherent with obtaining official confirmation through performing laboratory testing, it can take some weeks.

Digital epidemiology can be much quicker. Many of the digital data sources are collected real-time, with data being available pretty much as soon as it is collected. Mobile phone apps now exist allowing diagnosis at the point-of-care, literally at the patients bedside. Such apps can be accessed immediately by health officials meaning that notification of a potential problem occurs as soon as a potential case is spotted.

Sensitivity

In times past financial stockbrokers would use gut instinct on the trading floor to assess when stocks and shares might move up or down, and base their selling and buying decisions on this. Much depended on reading the body language of other traders. Those days are long gone. Instead share and stock dealing occurs behind a computer screen with data specialists monitoring data for the slightest indication that prices might go up or down. This illustrates how machine learning techniques are now being used to forecast future trends using the slightest deviations in share prices.

Other examples include programs to process blood samples allowing diagnosis to be made in minutes; previously such analysis could take days. The new mathematical methods allow slight alterations in case numbers which might be indicative of an outbreak to be detected before they become apparent to someone simply 'eyeballing' the data.

PROBLEMS AND ISSUES

Although digital epidemiology offers great potential, there are some potential problems which need consideration.

Ethics

Who owns the data? Key principles guiding the ethics of medical research include the requirement for informed consent from participants, the necessity for anonymity, and more recently the requirement to have access and control over data relating to oneself. Typically, medical research is strictly governed, with for example, ethical approval being required from a panel independent to the individual researchers before a study can proceed. The developments in digital epidemiology challenge these guiding principles in a number of ways.

- **Informed consent:** Often personal data is being collected without a participants knowledge. If I search on Google a record of this will be made and could be used later to generate data for Google Trends. Every time you make a mobile phone call, a record of it is made. Even if users are made aware such data is being collected, or permission is asked that it be used, this is often done vaguely. How many of us read the 'Terms and Conditions' box when it appears on the computer screen? Often we simply tick 'yes'. Do we know who our data is passed to? How would you feel if personal mobile phone records were used to infer your medical problems?

- **Anonymity:** Digital advancement mean it is easier than ever to make data anonymous. However equally as advanced is the ability of digital technology to overcome such attempts. It is now increasingly easy to cross reference between information sources, or use algorithms to 'guess' an individuals identity from a minimum of information. Ever opened up your email inbox to see adverts from holiday companies after searching for a weekend break? How do they know! The increasingly open nature of data means potentially personal information can become widely available and once released it is easily copied and distributed. Once out there, it can't be removed again.

- **Protected access:** A public health official working for a local governmental authority might be permitted to access personal information relating to individuals living in their area, including information on personal health issues and treatments. Such information could help guide provision of health care services and is potentially very useful. This access is usually limited to a few individuals. Such professionals are typically well trained, belong to a professional body which expects members to adhere to ethical standards, and have undergone vetting and training in data handling from their employer. But digital epidemiology challenges such safeguards. Often individuals where there is no such control have access to data.

Public health has always been a balance between an individuals right to autonomy and the need to protect the wider public by using personal information. The infectious nature of many conditions means that an individuals actions can have consequences for others. But where are the limits and what is acceptable and what not? Who decides?

COVID-19 highlighted some of the ethical challenges digital epidemiology faces. The COVID-19 pandemic was seen as an international emergency. But does this justify overriding personal rights for the public good? Mello and Wang (2020) describe some potentially problematic developments, providing the example of smartphones being used to classify Chinese citizens into risk groups which later affected their ability to move freely. Another example cited by Mello and Wang was from Taiwan, where potentially personally sensitive immigration records were linked with public health records.

Around the world a variety of contract tracing apps were developed during the COVID-19 pandemic which monitored the adherence of individuals to isolation and quarantine restrictions. The widespread use of such apps brought with them a requirement for personal details such as health status and geographical location, and the sharing of those to the wider community. Amnesty raised concerns about the use of this technology (Amnesty, 2020). In response to such concerns the European Data Protection Board released guidelines on the ethical use of data (EU, 2020). Kolassa et al. (2021) in a systematic review highlighted the problem that contact tracing apps that fully complied with privacy standards produced data of little public health interest. More useful data could be obtained only when privacy standards were relaxed.

Accountability

Traditionally, although those in public health roles might not be directly elected, they are at least often accountable to the public indirectly. For example, a local authority public health officer, often has an elected official nominally above them. This at least means there is some accountable control over such officials. It is obvious that such an official is working for the community, and with the ultimate purpose of aiding public health.

However, for an employee of a private technology who is working with health related data there is no such democratic control. Essentially the ultimate responsibility is to shareholders. The ultimate purpose is the generation of profit.

Accuracy and reliability

Traditional epidemiology relies on data generated through well established local, regional and national agencies (Velasco, 2018). Often well established and sometimes very detailed criteria exist to ensure that reporting of disease occurs in a standardized manner. Often data is verified. As Velasco (2018) noted, data is handled by professionals and can be considered of a high standard.

However, often criteria used in the collection of digital data is not as exact or thought through. Detailed standards do not exist, or cannot be obtained. There is no process of consultation and detailed thought. No external verification of data exists. Therefore the quality and accuracy of such data can often be uncertain.

Statistical concerns

Concerns exists as to the statistical validity of some of research produced using some types of digital data. Klingwort and Schnell (2020), in response to the development of mobile phone contact tracing apps, detailed a number of statistical concerns related to the data being used and the methods of working. A key issue raised is the making of inferences about the entire population, using uncertain samples from that population. For example, the old and infirm are less likely to use fitness trackers than young and fit people. Research making inferences for the entire population based on such data is likely to be incorrect. Similarly, mobile phone coverage varies across the age ranges, yet during the COVID-19 pandemic many researchers used data from mobile apps to determine population parameters such as number of infected people in the population and did not address this problem.

However, one can argue that although maybe the statistical rigour of many such studies may not be perfect, does this matter? Surely what is important to the health professional is that such research is useful on the ground. Can it usefully forecast future incidence rates or predict likely disease outbreaks?

A good example of potential issues related to reliability is demonstrated by the work of Cervellin et al. (2017), who examined data from Google Trends for various search terms and whether they were related to corresponding data in medical records. They examined a range of conditions, some of little media interest such as 'nose bleeding', 'renal colic' 'mushroom poisoning', and others which garnered much more media attention such as 'Ebola' and 'legionella'. The results suggested that media reports can greatly influence patterns seen on Google Trends. In some cases, determining the factors leading to trends in data could not be determined. For example, a rise in searching on mushroom poisoning coincided not unsurprisingly with the Autumn months when mushrooms are collected. The research emphasised that disentangling the reasons for trends in internet search data is difficult and more an art than a science.

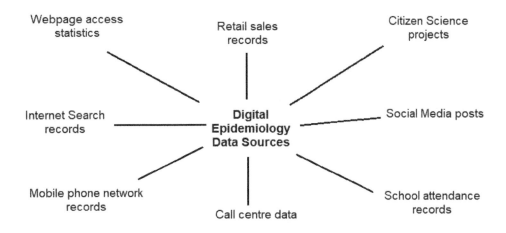

**Whether for work or play,
computers are at the centre of everyday life today.**

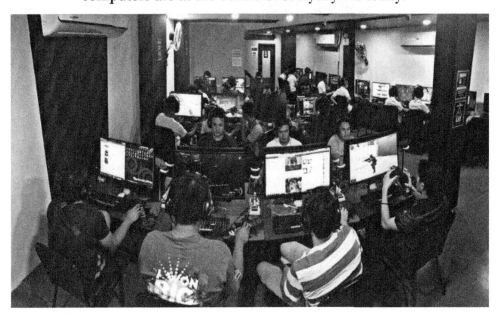

27

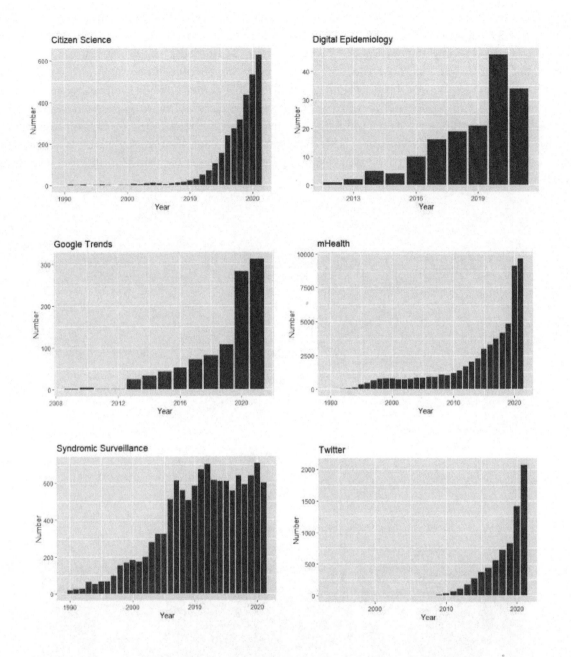

The steady rise of interest in digital epidemiology and related topics since 1990. Publications on key topics relevant to digital epidemiology. Results from PubMed searches for articles using the search terms 'citizen science', 'digital epidemiology', 'Google Trends', 'mHealth, 'syndromic surveillance' and 'Twitter'. To note, articles might not be all be medical or health related.

Where next?

A review by Park et al. (2018) examined digital epidemiology studies and looked at where the emphasis of them lay, what technologies they used, and which conditions they studied. It provided a good pointer as to where digital epidemiology currently is. The review identified a number of main topics that form most digital epidemiology studies. Of the 109 studies considered to be examples of 'digital epidemiology', most examine infectious diseases (58.7%), with the next largest proportion considering non-communicable diseases (29.4%), followed by mental health studies/substance abuse studies (8.3%). The most frequently used data source was internet search queries (52.3%), followed by social media posts (31.2%), then posts on web pages (11.9%). Fewer than 10% of the studies examined looked at web page accessing, digital images or used data from mobile phones. This review points the way future research could go. Image analysis is likely to grow in importance. Programming developments mean that this is becoming increasingly accurate. Additionally, the methods of doing this type of analysis are becoming more widely known. In conjunction with the analysis of images sent and received through mobile phones, this offers much potential for healthcare professionals in the future.

Another avenue with great potential interest is so called 'wearable' technology. These are devices that monitor personal body parameters such as heart rate and levels of activity. These are now well established consumer products and will become more commonly used as time progresses. Such technologies offer the potential to learn more about general trends occurring among populations that may be indicative of disease trends.

For example, Doherty et al. (2017) sent wrist worn devices, able to sense movement, to over 100,000 participants listed on the U.K. Biobank scheme. Participants wore these devices for seven days, with them automatically measuring participants level of activity. The results showed that those in older age ranges were less physically active, which is perhaps not surprising. However, they also indicate that women are more active that men, and that levels of activity remain similar regardless of day of week or season. These results are maybe more surprising. Although, this and similar studies highlight the potential of these devices, no study has yet used them for population based disease research. Potential avenues include measuring body temperature to assess whether it is elevated or not, which could possibly be indicative of influenza or other infectious disease.

Milinovich et al. (2014) emphasized that there was a plethora of retrospective studies, which demonstrated that digital data corresponded well with trends in disease. However, this only became apparent after the event. But there is a lack of prospective studies actually forecasting what will happen in the future. Also largely absent are studies evaluating previous digital epidemiology attempts, as highlighted by Zeeb (2020). As the sub discipline matures, emphasis on the effectiveness of digital epidemiology techniques should be strengthened.

The opening quote to this chapter comes from the Microsoft founder Bill Gates, and his Shattuck Lecture given in 2018 at the annual meeting of the Massachusetts Medical Society (Gates, 2018). This was later published in the New England Medical Journal. I selected this quote firstly because no one represents how the world has changed due to technological progress better than the totemic founder of Microsoft. Secondly, because the personal interest taken by Bill Gates in combating disease is widely known. The use of his personal wealth to combat disease through the Bill and Melinda Gates Foundation is laudable. The lecture he gave in 2018 proved eerily accurate, forecasting a global pandemic resulting in millions of deaths. It still remains valid today, the goal of the digital epidemiologist is now to prepare for the next pandemic, which will inevitably come.

REFERENCES

Andreu-Perez J, Poon CC, Merrifield RD, Wong ST, Yang GZ. Big data for health. *IEEE journal of biomedical and health informatics.* 2015;**19**(4):1193-208.

Amnesty International. Digital surveillance to fight COVID-19 can only be justified if it respects human rights. Amnesty International. 2020. Available at: https://www.amnesty.org/en/latest/news/2020/04/covid19-digital-surveillance-ngo/

Braithwaite I, Callender T, Bullock M, Aldridge RW. Automated and partly automated contact tracing: a systematic review to inform the control of COVID-19. *The lancet digital health.* 2020;**2**(11):e607-21.

British Medical Journal (BMJ). Epidemiology for the uninitiated. 2022. Available at: bmj.com/about-bmj/resources-readers/publications/epidemiology-uninitiated/1-what-epidemiology#chapters

Brownstein JS, Freifeld CC, Reis BY, Mandl KD. Surveillance Sans Frontieres: internet-based emerging infectious disease intelligence and the HealthMap project. *Plos medicine.* 2008;**5**(7):e151.

Brownstein JS, Freifeld CC, Madoff LC. Digital disease detection—harnessing the Web for public health surveillance. *New England journal of medicine.* 2009;**360**:2153.

Cervellin G, Comelli I, Lippi G. Is Google Trends a reliable tool for digital epidemiology? Insights from different clinical settings. *Journal of epidemiology and global health.* 2017;**7**(3):185-9.

Davenport TH, Patil DJ. Data scientist. *Harvard business review.* 2012;**90**(5):70-6.

Doherty A, Jackson D, Hammerla N, Plötz T, Olivier P, Granat MH, White T, Van Hees VT, Trenell MI, Owen CG, Preece SJ. Large scale population assessment of physical activity using wrist worn accelerometers: the UK biobank study. *Plos one.* 2017;**12**(2):e0169649.

Eckhoff PA, Tatem AJ. Digital methods in epidemiology can transform disease control. *International health.* 2015;**7**(2):77-78.

Eckmanns T, Hempel L. DELSI—digital epidemiology and its ethical, legal and social implications. Call for Abstracts by the Robert-Koch-Institute. 2015.

European Union (EU). Regulation (EU) 2016/679 of the European Parliament and of the Council of 27 April 2016 on the protection of natural persons with regard to the processing of personal data and on the free movement of such data, and repealing Directive 95/46/EC (General Data Protection Regulation). Eur-Lex. 2016. Available online at: https://eur-lex.europa.eu/eli/reg/2016/679/oj

Eysenbach G. Infodemiology: The epidemiology of (mis)information. *American journal of medicine.* 2002;**113**(9):763-5.

Gates B. Innovation for pandemics. *New England journal of medicine.* 2018;**378**(22):2057-60.

Ginsberg J, Mohebbi MH, Patel RS, Brammer L, Smolinski MS, Brilliant L. Detecting influenza epidemics using search engine query data. *Nature.* 2009;**457**:1012-14.

Henning KJ. What is syndromic surveillance? *MMWR morbity and mortality weekly report.* 2004, **53** (Suppl): 5-11.

Iavindrasana J, Cohen G, Depeursinge A, Müller H, Meyer R, Geissbuhler A. Clinical data mining: a review. *Yearbook of medical informatics.* 2009;**18**(01):121-33.

IBM. What is Data Mining? 2022. Available at: www.ibm.com/cloud/learn/data-mining

IBM. Big Data Analytics. 2022. Available at: www.ibm.com/analytics/big-data-analytics

Klingwort J, Schnell R. Critical limitations of digital epidemiology. *Survey and research methods.* 2020;**14**(2):95-101.

Kolasa K, Mazzi F, Leszczuk-Czubkowska E, Zrubka Z, Péntek M. State of the art in adoption of contact tracing apps and recommendations regarding privacy protection and public health: Systematic review. *JMIR mHealth and uHealth*. 2021;**9**(6):e23250.

Lee CH, Yoon HJ. Medical big data: promise and challenges. *Kidney research and clinical practice*. 2017;**36**(1):3.

Liu W, Beltagui A, Ye S. Accelerated innovation through repurposing: exaptation of design and manufacturing in response to COVID-19. *R&D management*. 2021;**51**(4):410-26.

Menni C, Valdes AM, Freidin MB, Sudre CH, Nguyen LH, Drew DA, Ganesh S, Varsavsky T, Cardoso MJ, El-Sayed Moustafa JS, Visconti A. Real-time tracking of self-reported symptoms to predict potential COVID-19. *Nature medicine*. 2020;**26**(7):1037-40.

Mello MM, Wang CJ. Ethics and governance for digital disease surveillance. *Science*. 2020;**368**(6494):951-4.

Milinovich GJ, Williams GM, Clements AC, Hu W. internet-based surveillance systems for monitoring emerging infectious diseases. *Lancet infectious diseases*. 2014;**14**(2):160-8.

National Health Service (NHS). Digital Annual Report. 2020 to 2021. Accessed from: digital.nhs.uk/about-nhs-digital/corporate-information-and-documents/nhs-digital-s-annual-reports-and-accounts/nhs-digital-annual-report-and-accounts-2020-21

Nuffield Trust. NHS 111 data. Available at: www.nuffieldtrust.org.uk/resource/nhs-111#background

Office for National Statistics (ONS). Internet Access: Households and Individuals.. Annual reports. 2020. Available at: www.ons.gov.uk/peoplepopulationandcommunity/householdcharacteristics/homeinternetandsocialmediausage/bulletins/internetaccesshouseholdsandindividuals/2020

Park HA, Jung H, On J, Park SK, Kang H. Digital epidemiology: use of digital data collected for non-epidemiological purposes in epidemiological studies. *Healthcare informatics research*. 2018;**24**(4):253-62.

Salathé M, Bengtsson L, Bodnar TJ, Brewer DD, Brownstein JS, Buckee C, Campbell EM, Cattuto C, Khandelwal S, Mabry PL, Vespignani A. Digital epidemiology. 2012.

Salathé M, Freifeld CC, Mekaru SR, Tomasulo AF, Brownstein JS. Influenza A (H7N9) and the importance of digital epidemiology. *New England journal of medicine*. 2013;**369**(5):401-404.

Salathé M. Digital epidemiology: what is it, and where is it going? *Life sciences, society and policy*. 2018;**14**:1-8.

World Health Organization (WHO). WHO guideline: recommendations on digital interventions for health system strengthening. Geneva: World Health Organization; 2019.

World Health Organization (WHO). World malaria report. 2021. ISBN: 978 92 4 004049 6.

Velasco E. Disease detection, epidemiology and outbreak response: the digital future of public health practice. *Life sciences, society and policy*. 2018;**14**:7.

Zeeb H, Pigeot I, Schüz B. Digital Public Health – Ein Überblick. *Bundesgesundheitsblatt*. 2020;**63**:137-144.

DATA SCIENCE AND
DISEASE SURVEILLANCE

It's all just a little bit of history repeating

Shirley Bassey, Song lyrics.

The concept of 'data science' as a distinct subject is relatively modern. The name was being used in the early 1980's, and has been attributed to various people (Wu, 1985). Despite this, its roots are deep. Data science draws heavily on statistics, a subject which has a long history. Many of the methods being used in modern data science are thus based upon ones which are well established. Many methods considered cutting edge are simply variations on traditional practises. Hence, the choice of opening quote.

Imagine a scientist wanting to investigate whether the incidence of a particular condition is increasing or decreasing within a particular geographical area, and which environmental factors might be influencing this. Obtaining data on the number of people affected by this condition over a period of historical time might be relatively easy. But once you have this data what should you do with it next? Obtaining the data required is only the first initial stage of the scientific process.

As important as obtaining data is knowing how to manage it once you have it. A vital part of the scientific process is observation. Thus an important first task for the disease epidemiologist is to examine the data and see what it shows. Are there missing values? What are the averages? When does it peak? When is it lowest? What strikes you about it? Once the investigator has a good 'feel' for the data, then decisions need to be made on how to handle it to investigate the research question you are interested in.

The opening chapter described the digital revolution that has occurred over the past 30 years and the ways this has impacted on epidemiology. Much of the rest of this book looks at the new sources of data that this digital revolution has opened up. However, before examining these, it first makes sense to look at how digital developments have impacted how disease scientists analyse the data they have. How has data analysis changed in the past 30 years? These developments are so numerous it is impossible to be comprehensive here; instead I provide a pot-pourri of some examples of new, improved or simply popular methods.

Big data in public health and disease surveillance

It has been known for some time that big data concepts are of importance in public health and disease surveillance. The most basic statistic is simply the number of cases of a particular condition over time. This might seem a relatively straightforward piece of data to collect. It can be obtained from a number of sources. For example, Simonsen et al. (2016) lists death certificates, hospital admissions, emergency departments, outpatient visits, and results from laboratory testing, all as potential sources of this information. These can all be considered as 'official' sources. However, identifying potential sources is one thing, deciding which is the best and most accurate is another.

What about non-official informal sources that might show the number of possible cases or at least provide an indication of them? As the following chapters will illustrate, such sources are rapidly increasing in number. Such data might include medication sales information, calls made to health hotlines, internet search results, and even social media mentions.

Whatever the source, the size of such datasets is increasingly large. Just think about data related to pharmacy sales; there might be dozens of pharmacists, each selling a multitude of products, over many weeks and months.

Where does disease surveillance 'big data' come from?

'Formal'	'Informal'
Official case number data from public health agencies	Internet searches
Death certificates	Social media posts
Hospital admission or medical practitioner visits	Telephone calls to medical hotlines
Sentinel medical practitioner data	Sales data

The ability to collect data relating to disease has increased. Health records are now increasingly being held electronically, which greatly facilitates data management and collaboration. For example, it is now much easier to establish a sentinel system based upon medical practitioners serving local communities than was previously the case. A sentinel surveillance system is where a small selection of information sources are used to gather data on disease occurrence, in the hope that this reflects the wider trends in the populations being studied.

Previously recorded data on health matters would be paper based, with data being submitted to public health officials perhaps on a weekly basis. Many datasets provided in the U.K. are provided on a monthly and sometimes even a quarterly basis. For example, data on the number of cases of various zoonotic conditions is published only every three months. Even the publication of data on notifiable conditions is released in the U.K. only on a weekly basis.

Systems can now be automated with data being collected as part of standard recording procedures, then sent for central processing electronically, at intervals much quicker than was previously the case. GitHub provides an example of how easy it is to share data now; this resource provides a platform for data sharing. Health related datasets are often placed upon GitHub sites by healthcare researchers.

DATA SCIENCE METHODS IN DISEASE SCIENCE: EXAMPLES

Following are a selection of methods and techniques that have developed as a consequence of improved computing power. They demonstrate some of the ways researchers are now studying disease.

Disease diagnosis using machine learning

A key requisite for epidemiologists is that diseases are diagnosed correctly and accurately. Machine learning techniques have helped improve the initial diagnosis of disease. There are many examples. Just to provide one, the study by Sun et al. (2017) used measurements of respiration, heart rate and facial temperatures to classify individuals at risk of influenza using neural networking and fuzzy clustering. Another by Go et al. (2018), used machine learning algorithms to detect red blood corpuscles infected with malaria. There are many such studies.

A currently hot topic for researchers is image processing. Much medical diagnosis is based upon the interpretation of images. It turns out that machine learning can be as effective as the most well trained physician. Plus computers don't get tired! Methods such as convolutional neural networks are able to 'scan' images and 'decide' if the signs of a particular condition are present within an image or not.

The website Kaggle shows how easy it is to share data, ideas and techniques today. Kaggle is predominately a coding site, with the emphasis being on machine learning techniques. But anyone can take part. The diagnosis of disease is a common theme for competition, discussion and code sharing on Kaggle. For example, during the early phases of the COVID-19 pandemic a competition was run asking teams to forecast COVID-19 spread for different regions on the world (Kaggle, 2020).

Disease surveillance using machine learning

Machine learning has also been used directly for disease surveillance. Sadilek et al. (2018) developed a machine learning model entitled FINDER, which used data from web searching to determine the location of potential food poisoning cases. They examined the search terms used by those who had visited restaurants to determine whether they were suffering the symptoms of food poisoning. This information was then used to send food inspectors to particular restaurants. The ones identified by FINDER were over three time more likely to be deemed unsafe after such visits than those being visited routinely at random.

Another example is provided by Luo et al. (2015). This study used data on the socio-demographic features of respondents to the American Community Survey. They used machine learning to predict the prevalence of six non-communicable diseases including obesity, diabetes, high blood pressure, and a range of cardiovascular diseases. The methods used included machine learning techniques such as random forests, LASSO regression and stepwise regression.

A number of studies have compared machine learning approaches to more traditional methods. Tessmer et al. (2018) compared three machine learning methods: Multi layer perception, convolutional neural networks, and long short term memory (LSTM) recurrent neural network models, against more traditional compartmental SEIR models, and studied the ability to forecast a range of infectious diseases. Zhang et al. (2022) compared traditional ARIMA times series modelling with more modern neural networking models in the forecasting of dengue fever.

Regression analyses for disease surveillance

Regression is a mathematical method to study the relationship between an outcome or response variable and one or more dependant variables or predictors. Essentially, the line of best fit is placed between the variables being examined. Regression can be used to find the importance of variables and to make forecasts as to likely expected values that might occur in the future. It assumes that the variables being examined are related to each other. The most basic and traditionally used method was simple linear regression; a straight line is used and placed where the distance of each point from the line is a minimum.

When thinking about machine learning one might think of highly complex techniques involving complex algorithms or dense mathematical equations. However, actually regression is an important machine learning technique itself, despite its simplicity. In fact regression is one of the most widespread machine learning techniques there is.

As computing power increased and statistical analyses became easier to perform, more complex forms of regression became more common. These include generalized linear models, which examine whether data follows a Poisson, binomial or negative binomial distribution. These are particularly useful when studying disease as often the distribution of cases rarely fits a normal Gaussian pattern. Other methods of performing regression include using time series modelling for regression purposes, such as using standard ARMA or ARIMA models (See section below). Favoured by machine learning fans are specialised methods such as XGBoost. Increasingly common are methods based upon neural networks, such as recurrent neural networks and LSTM. Techniques for overcoming some of the limitations of basic linear regression have become more common such as ridge regression.

The use of regression for disease prediction purposes is common, and examples can easily be found in the scientific literature. Use of regression techniques is increasing in popularity. As an example Chen et al. (2018) used LASSO regression to examine the influence of climate on a number of diseases including chickenpox, dengue, and malaria for countries including Japan, Thailand, and Singapore. They were able to make short term forecasts four weeks in advance using this technique.

Scavuzzo et al. (2018) used various machine learning methods to model reproduction parameters of *Aedes ægypti* mosquitoes in Argentina. These mosquitoes are the main vector for chikungunya, dengue fever, and the Zika virus. They used a range of weather variables obtained from satellite data. Compared to standard linear modelling the new machine learning techniques proved best, with nearest neighbour regression (NNR) being the most accurate.

Some machine learning methods of performing regression analyses.

ARMA	LSTM
ARIMA	Poisson based regression
ANN	Neural networking
LASSO	Random forests
Ridge regression	XGBoost

Classification and clustering for disease surveillance

Another task machine learning techniques excel at is classification. In classification the decision is made as to which group an individual belongs to. Classification uses the features made available to it to predict the chances that an event will occur or not. This is an example of supervised learning; the outcome is known, and the statistical program must decide into which categories particular data points belong. For example, at the most simplest, will someone develop a condition or not?

A popular and well known form of classification often used in the health sciences is logistic regression. Advanced computing means there are now a wide array of other classification techniques; decision trees, random forests, support vector machines and neural networks.

Unlike classification, clustering is unsupervised. The outcomes are not provided; the algorithm has to decide on these itself. Clustering is basically deciding whether data belongs into groups, and then making the decision as to which groups each data point belongs to. This is decided using distance metrics. Example techniques often used include K-means clustering and principal components analysis.

As an example of classification, Balasaravanan and Prakash (2018) used neural networking with data on a range of patient characteristics to determine which ones had dengue fever.

Time series analysis and disease forecasting

Time series analysis can be described as the study of how events change over time. A time series is simply a series of data points collected at different time periods. Time series are ubiquitous, and once you start looking for them they are everywhere. A classic example is the daily price of stocks and shares over a year.

Time series analysis is not a new subject. People have tried to understand how and why things alter over time for centuries. However, the awareness that time series analysis is a discipline in its own right is more recent. Many of the specific techniques currently popular were developed in the early to mid 20th century. The availability of big data and modern statistical computing has revitalised this field. Calculations which were tedious and time consuming can now be performed in seconds on a home laptop.

The study of time series is of particularly interest in epidemiology. After all the most basic statistics in epidemiology is the record of the number of cases of a disease or condition. Time series analysis helps in understanding how patterns in disease change over time. For example, it is now easy to separate different aspects of a time series automatically. This is known as time series decomposition, which teases out seasonal, underlying trend and random components contained within the time series, with one of the most popular methods being the Seasonal Trend Decomposition using LOESS – known as STL (Cleveland et al. 1990).

Another key task for disease epidemiologists is forecasting. Obviously, a disease biologist wants to estimate the potential future number of cases. Again, many of the methods used today have a long history, but the difference is that they are increasingly easy to implement. Traditional forecasting methods include simple autoregressive models, where future values depend on previous ones. Also common are the classic Box-Jenkins ARIMA models. Essentially, ARIMA is modelling using a combination of autoregressive, trending and moving average components. Despite its simplicity ARIMA often proves very effective, often more effective than other more complex techniques. Over the past decade a wide array of much more computationally intense methods have gained favour. These include decision trees, random forests and neural networking models. But often these are no better than the traditional techniques.

Early examples where ARIMA was used for disease purposes include Choi and Thacker (1981), who used these methods to study influenza. Helfenstein (1986) used ARIMA to examine chicken pox and mumps. These techniques have become increasingly popular to model disease incidence as knowledge of how to implement them has become more widespread. Use of these time series techniques is now commonplace and reached a peak during the COVID-19 pandemic; a Google Scholar search on 'COVID-19' and 'ARIMA' produced 18,200 results in mid 2022.

Making forecasts is now quick and easy to do on a home personal computer: Below is a forecast for measles for England and Wales using a seasonal ARIMA model with components (0,1,2)(0,1,2)(52). This was produced using data on reported cases from the Notification of Infectious Diseases (NOIDS) dataset for England and Wales from June 2020 to January 2021.

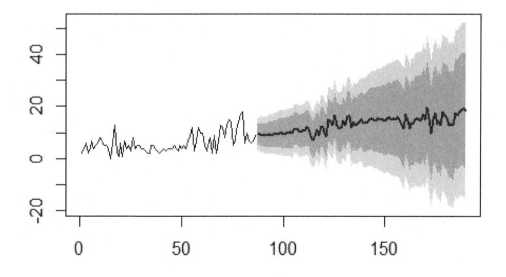

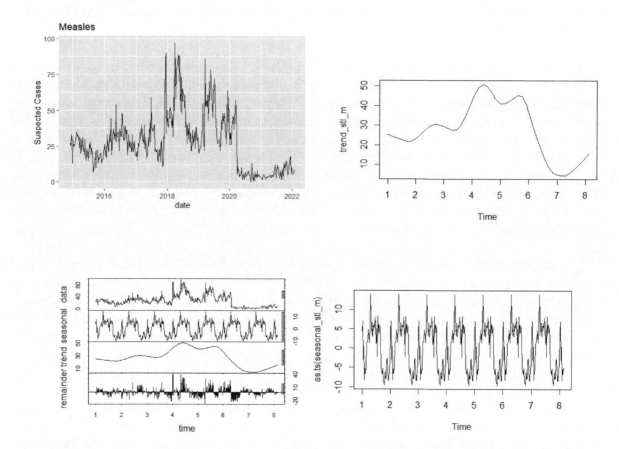

Above: How modern computing allows time series to be examined. Here, top left, the weekly number of suspected cases of measles reported by various healthcare professionals to public health England/Health Security Agency as part of Notification of Infectious Diseases 'NOIDS'. Data is weekly from 2014 to 2022. Modern programming allows break down, 'decomposition', of the time series. Here, this is done using the 'STL' method, which breaks it into the underlying trend, seasonal affects, and random effects. Top left shows the complete time series, top right shows the left underlying trend, bottom right shows the seasonal trend, bottom left shows each of these. This allows features to be studied. Note the fall in trend coinciding with Spring 2020. The clear seasonal nature of suspected cases is clear from the seasonal plot at bottom right.

Agent based modelling

Imagine a single person harbouring an infectious disease as they go about their everyday life. They catch the bus, stand in the queue at the coffee shop, catch a full lift up to the office. They then sit amongst their work colleagues in a small meeting room. All the time they are potentially transmitting the pathogen they harbour to others. Wouldn't it be good if we could model such interactions and how they influence disease transmission?

Agent based modelling allows you to do exactly that. Instead of looking at disease from a population based perspective, it looks at it at the individual scale and looks at how individual differences in state or behaviour influence overall progression of a disease at the population level. The effect on the population is considered as being the result of the influence of individuals each possessing different properties (Auchincloss and Diez Roux, 2008). Individuals, known as 'agents', move through a virtual landscape coming into contact with other 'agents' that may or may not harbour a disease, and who possess different properties, such as the chance of becoming infected.

This allows researchers to investigate the course infectious diseases take under different scenarios. For example, the influence of pathogens with different levels of virulence can be examined, or the effect of different levels of vaccine uptake, or the influence of agents with different characteristics. For example, 'super spreaders' are individuals who when infected go on to transmit their pathogen to a large number of others. Agent based modelling allows the influence of agents with different such levels of 'sociability' to be assessed.

A well cited and early example of agent-based modelling was the study by Halloran et al. (2002). This study used agent-based modelling to examine what would happen if smallpox was released into a naïve population. The study looked at the difference mass vaccination would have compared to more targeted vaccination. It also examined the influence of residual immunity present in older generations that had been vaccinated against smallpox.

Another good example where agent-based modelling has been used is Kumar et al. (2015). They simulated an epidemic of influenza, similar in nature to H1N1 influenza, and the effect of agents of different socio-economic level. They thus showed that there was a connection between poverty and influenza attack rate.

GIS and the spatial analysis of disease

Examining the spatial distribution of disease is not new. One of the first topics possibly every student studying epidemiology or disease science learns about is how the Victorian pioneer Jon Snow mapped cholera cases around drinking wells around Broad Street, London. He thus determined the water borne nature of the condition, arguably establishing epidemiology as a science at the same time.

The process of mapping disease has advanced considerably in recent decades. Epidemiologists are obviously interested in how disease cases are distributed spatially and what could be causing such a distribution. The simplest form of spatial analysis is simply to plot cases of disease on a map. Simply visualizing such data allows patterns and distributions to be seen that can not be identified by simply reading a list of numbers or written locations. However, it is not only disease cases themselves that are spatial in nature, but a number of related factors influencing disease occurrence such as environmental factors like weather or pollution levels.

As mentioned in Chapter 1, Geographic Information Systems (GIS) became widely available from the late 1990's and have changed spatial epidemiology beyond recognition. Now examining the spatial nature of disease is in the scope of every epidemiologist. Cromley (2003) provides an excellent review of early GIS based studies examining public health issues and disease. Early examples include mapping of arsenic concentrations in water from wells in Western Texas (Hudak et al. 2000), and a study of carcinogens in domestic water wells in Maryland which identified the areas of greatest risk (Bolton and Hayes, 1999).

GIS has proved of much use in the study of vector borne conditions, where it allows the mapping of vectors or hosts. One example of this is the study of tick abundance by Guerra et al. (2002) where 138 different sites were studied. The ticks present on small mammals were assessed as well as the abundance of questing ticks in the environment, in order to study which environmental variables influenced tick abundance most. Another example is from soil helminths, which transmit a range of parasitic conditions. Magalhães et al. (2011) examined the influence different water and sanitation measures had on the burden of helminth infestation in school children.

Hay et al. (2009) used data from over 7,953 surveys of the malaria protozoan blood parasite *Plasmodium falciparum* to model where malaria was endemic across the globe. Such work has helped understand malaria distributions better. The Global Malaria Atlas provides maps related to malaria prevalence and a range of intervention measures, allowing a unique perspective on the global battle against malaria. It is obvious how such information can help better understand malaria distribution, and help in effective management and resource allocation against this pernicious condition.

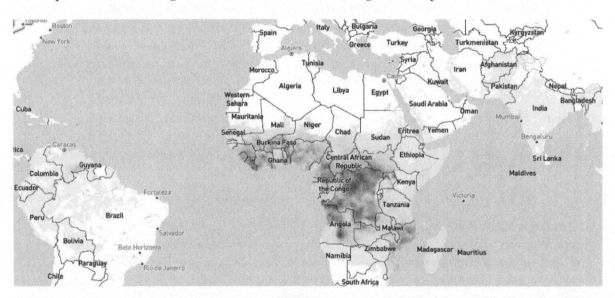

An example map from the Malaria Atlas Project. This is principally funded by the Bill and Melinda Gates foundation. This shows the presence of the *Plasmodium falciparum* blood parasite in 2020. See Hay et al. (2009) for an earlier map of malaria prevalence. Image from: https://malariaatlas.org

REFERENCES

Auchincloss AH, Diez Roux AV. A new tool for epidemiology: The usefulness of dynamic-agent models in understanding place effects on health. *American journal of epidemiology.* 2008;**168**(1):1-8.

Balasaravanan K, Prakash M. Detection of dengue disease using artificial neural network based classification technique. *International journal of engineering and technology.* 2018;**7**(1.3):13-5.

Bolton DW, Hayes MA. Pilot Study of Carcinogens in Well Water in Anne Arundel County, Maryland. Open File Report. MD geol. surv. Baltimore. 1999.

Chen Y, Chu CW, Chen MI, Cook AR. The utility of lasso-based models for real time forecasts of endemic infectious diseases: a cross country comparison *Journal of biomedical informatics.* 2018;**81**:16-30.

Choi K, Thacker SB. An evaluation of influenza mortality surveillance, 1962–1979: I. Time series forecasts of expected pneumonia and influenza deaths. *American journal of epidemiology.* 1981;**113**(3):215-26.

Cleveland RB, Cleveland WS, McRae JE, Terpenning I. STL: a seasonal trend decomposition procedure based on loess. *Journal of official statistics.* 1990; 3-73.

Cromley EK. GIS and disease. *Annual review of public health.* 2003;**24**:7.

Go T, Kim JH, Byeon H, Lee SJ. Machine learning-based in-line holographic sensing of unstained malaria-infected red blood cells. *Journal of biophotonics.* 2018;**11**(9):e201800101.

Guerra M, Walker E, Jones C, Paskewitz S, Cortinas MR, Stancil A, Beck L, Bobo M, Kitron U. Predicting the risk of Lyme disease: habitat suitability for *Ixodes scapularis* in the North Central United States. *Emerging infectious diseases.* 2002;**8**:289-97.

Halloran ME, Longini IM, Nizam A, Yang Y. Containing bioterrorist smallpox. *Science.* 2002;**298**(5597):1428-32.

Hay SI, Battle KE, Pigott DM, Smith DL, Moyes CL, Bhatt S, Brownstein JS, Collier N, Myers MF, George DB. Global mapping of infectious disease. *Philosophical transactions of the royal society of London B: Biological sciences.* 2013;**368**:20120250.

Hay SI, Guerra CA, Gething PW, Patil AP, Tatem AJ, Noor AM, Kabaria CW, Manh BH, Elyazar IR, Brooker S, Smith DL. A world malaria map: *Plasmodium falciparum* endemicity in 2007. *Plos medicine.* 2009;**6**: e1000048.

Helfenstein U. Box-Jenkins modelling of some viral infectious diseases. *Statistics in medicine.* 1986;**5**(1):37-47.

Hudak PF. Distribution and sources of arsenic in the southern High Plains Aquifer, Texas, USA. *Journal of environmental science and health.* 2000;**A35**:899-913

Kaggle. COVID10 Global Forecasting challenge. 2020. Available at: www.kaggle.com/competitions/covid19-global-forecasting-week-1/overview

Kumar S, Piper K, Galloway DD, Hadler JL, Grefenstette JJ. Is population structure sufficient to generate area-level inequalities in influenza rates? An examination using agent-based models. *BMC public health.* 2015;**15**:947.

Luo W, Nguyen T, Nichols M, Tran T, Rana S, Gupta S, Phung D, Venkatesh S, Allender S. Is demography destiny? Application of machine learning techniques to accurately predict population health outcomes from a minimal demographic dataset. *Plos one.* 2015;**10**(5):e0125602.

Sadilek A, Caty S, DiPrete L, Mansour R, Schenk T, Bergtholdt M, Jha A, Ramaswami P, Gabrilovich E. Machine-learned epidemiology: real-time detection of foodborne illness at scale. *Npj digital medicine.* 2018;**1**(1):36.

Scavuzzo JM, Trucco F, Espinosa M, Tauro CB, Abril M, Scavuzzo CM, Frery AC. Modeling dengue vector population using remotely sensed data and machine learning. *Acta tropica.* 2018;**185**:167-175.

Sun G, Matsui T, Hakozaki Y, Abe S. An infectious disease/fever screening radar system which stratifies higher--risk patients within ten seconds using a neural network and the fuzzy grouping method. *Journal of infection.* 2015;**70**(3):230-6.

Tessmer HL, Ito K, Omori R. Can machines learn respiratory virus epidemiology?: A comparative study of likelihood-free methods for the estimation of epidemiological dynamics. *Frontiers in microbiology.* 2018;**9**:343.

Zhang R, Song H, Chen Q, Wang Y, Wang S, Li Y. Comparison of ARIMA and LSTM for prediction of hemorrhagic fever at different time scales in China. *Plos one.* 2022;**17**(1):e0262009.

3

HOW TO DEVELOP A SYNDROMIC SURVEILLANCE SYSTEM

Coughs and sneezes spread diseases

US Public Health Service. Slogan in response
to 'Spanish Flu', 1918.

Do you know that tickle in your throat or that feeling of fatigue, that tells you that you are not 100 percent today? An illness rarely develops instantaneously. Instead symptoms can insidiously develop over several days. Most of us only turn to a medical professional when we are really quite poorly and realize that we can not treat ourselves, or do not know how to.

This is essentially the principle of syndromic surveillance. It is the study of symptoms and ailments indicative of illness, before a diagnosis is made and cases appears in official records. By tracking when symptoms start to develop within a population before being officially recognized, possible outbreaks can be anticipated and measures put in place to mediate problems that might occur.

Defining syndromic surveillance

That there was no consensus as to a standard definition for syndromic surveillance was highlighted by Katz et al. (2011). In this review over 30 different definitions for syndromic surveillance were identified. There is also confusion over the name. Henning (2004) listed a number of alternatives which are used, including 'outbreak detection systems' and 'early warning systems'. He noted that despite other more recent suggestions, the name syndromic surveillance had persisted.

A commonly cited definition is the one provided by Mandl et al. (2004). This is a very broad definition, less concerned with the utilization of symptoms, and more concerned with early identification of disease outbreaks. It defined syndromic surveillance as:

> Methods relying on detection of clinical case features that are discernible before confirmed diagnoses are made.

After this opening definition, it was then emphasized that syndromic surveillance is based on 'behavioural patterns, symptoms, signs, or laboratory findings'. The identification of bio-terrorist threats is accorded great importance in the text by Mandl (2004). Perhaps this is not surprising, given that it was written only a few years after the September 11 attacks of 2001. Another commonly used definition is that from Henning (2004):

> The fundamental objective of syndromic surveillance is to identify illness clusters early, before diagnoses are confirmed and reported to public health agencies, and to mobilize a rapid response, thereby reducing morbidity and mortality.

Although many definitions concentrate on the fact that syndromic surveillance allows the early identification of potential disease outbreaks, many also mention that it often uses non-conventional data sources, such as internet search records or data on ambulance calls outs. Katz (2011) proposed a classification, identifying two main types of syndromic surveillance; one a specific form based on a specific set of well defined symptoms, and a second more general type which instead looked for more general indications that an outbreak was occurring.

In this chapter, syndromic surveillance is used in the sense of attempting to identify trends in a particular disease or condition by examining a well defined list of symptoms related to that condition.

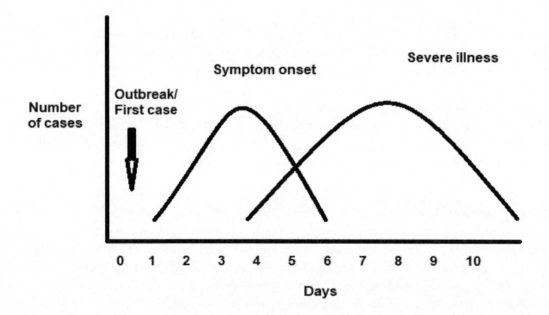

The fundamental principle behind syndromic surveillance: Symptoms appear before severe illness develops. Adapted from Henning (2004).

The development of syndromic surveillance

Is increased interest in syndromic surveillance related to advances in digital technology? The development and invention of many of the data sources mentioned later in this book have been used in the establishment of syndromic surveillance systems. The development of these data sources has fuelled interest in syndromic surveillance.

Before the availability of many of these new data sources, there was often no indication of what symptoms people were experiencing before they actually attended a medical centre and these were recorded. Additionally, advances now mean that records can be shared much easier and quicker than before. This is essential for syndromic surveillance to work. Syndromic surveillance relies on speed; records indicative of symptoms and potential illness need to reach epidemiologists quicker than those collected through traditional record processing do.

Interest in syndromic surveillance began to develop in the 1990's. As indicated above, an important impetus in the development of such systems was the desire to spot bio-terrorist attacks in the wake of the 2001 anthrax and September 11 terrorist attacks in the U.S. However, probably more important were the new avenues opened up by technological progress at the time.

DEVELOPING SYNDROMIC SURVEILLANCE

How do you develop a syndromic surveillance system? Mandl et al. (2004) outlined the key decisions and steps required in the setting up of such a system.

- **Which diseases? Which conditions?:** Which diseases are going to be examined? Which can be examined in this way?

- **Which syndromes are going to be studied?** What range of symptoms potentially indicate cases of the disease being studied. Where can this information be obtained from?

- **What type of data are required?** Which data sources are best suited to the proposed syndromic system? Also, which statistical techniques are going to be used to determine when an outbreak is occurring?

Which diseases? Which conditions?

Some conditions lend themselves better to early detection than others. Conditions where there is a long period before severe symptoms develop are better suited for syndromic surveillance. Where initial symptoms become evident early on, well before severe illness develops, this means there is time for the condition to be potentially spotted. Also helpful is if the early symptoms are particularly distinct. For example, in early infections with the tick-borne condition Lyme disease a characteristic rash often appears. This is known as a 'bull's eye rash' because of its distinctive circular shape with pale middle. Such a clear symptom can be easily spotted, recorded and tracked.

However, other conditions are not so suitable for syndromic surveillance. This may be because they are difficult to diagnose. Think of the respiratory condition pertussis, often referred to as whooping cough. This is a infectious bacterial condition, which in children can result in a distinctive 'whooping' cough. But this cough is not always evident. In adults pertussis may present as a persistent hacking cough, not dissimilar to a smoker's cough or those associated with long lasting colds we all have experience of. As the figure below illustrates, there are a number of potential causative agents behind such a cough, and infectious diseases are only some of them. Without microbiological testing it is difficult to determine definitely that a cough is being caused by pertussis.

Also important to bear in mind are the number of people affected by a particular condition and potential cost benefits to a healthcare service of spotting increases in a condition. Influenza is of great cost both in terms of lives lost and the financial burden it causes to health services. Many thousands of people are affected by influenza in the U.K. each year. Therefore being able to anticipate when peaks in influenza cases will occur would be of great benefit. However, this is arguably not one of the best conditions for syndromic surveillance from a symptom point of view. The symptoms experienced by those suffering influenza vary considerably on an individual basis. Additionally many of the early symptoms mirror those of other less serious conditions such as the common cold. Despite these problems, great effort goes into forecasting influenza peaks because of the great benefits such forecasts offer.

Scale is also a potential problem. Much early interest in syndromic surveillance was in spotting bioterrorist attacks such as an anthrax attack. However, the postal attacks in 2001 in the U.S. resulted in 22 cases. Spotting such an attack among a population of millions is difficult. The data used for syndromic surveillance is often 'noisy' with unexpected spikes and falls and rises. Spotting potential small scale outbreaks amongst such noisy data is difficult.

Symptoms and syndromes

Because of these problems most emphasis has gone into examining a suite of symptoms that may indicate general levels of a specific condition, instead of looking for changes in the occurrence of a single very exact symptom. A syndrome is the name for a collection of symptoms associated with a particular condition. Fricker (2013) defined this as:

> A syndrome is a set of symptoms or conditions that occur together and suggest the presence of a certain disease or an increased chance of developing the disease.

Thus, important in establishing syndromic surveillance is selecting an appropriate list of symptoms to study for the condition one is interested in (Reingold et al. 2003).

As an example, WHO (2001) recognizes five syndrome categories:
- haemorrhagic fever syndrome
- respiratory syndrome
- diarrhoeal syndrome
- jaundice syndrome
- neurological syndrome

What type of data is required?

The subsequent chapters illustrate some potential data sources that can be used for syndromic surveillance, and provide some examples where such data has already been successfully used. Which type of data is used depends on what is available, and which is best suited for the system being established. This could well be condition specific.

Potentially very useful to those wishing to establish syndromic surveillance systems are ICD-10 codes (recently updated to ICD-11). These provide some standardization of symptoms and potential complaints. However, an issue with the use of these is that most typically such codes are only allocated once a diagnosis has already been made, or at least suspected. Thus strictly speaking, a syndromic surveillance system using these is not really syndromic. An example of a system using ICD codes is the ESSENCE system, Electronic Surveillance System for Early Notification of Community-based Epidemics, which is introduced below.

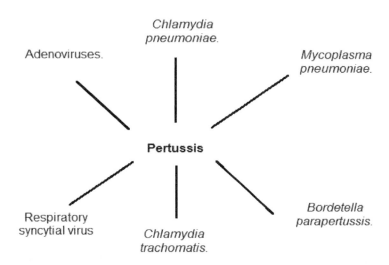

The problem of differentials: here a list of infectious causes of a cough that present similarly to pertussis. Taken from: What else could it be? Whooping Cough. Clinical Knowledge Summaries (NICE, 2022). To note, these are only possible infectious causes of a cough, a long list of chronic conditions also result in a cough. This illustrates the potential problem of using a single symptom when attempting to track a specific condition.

Analysing data: spotting abnormalities, detecting changes
Obtaining potentially useful data is one thing, but how will an outbreak be detected once you have it? As mentioned epidemiological data is often 'noisy' in nature. It does not remain steady and level, there are occasional increases and dips, unexpected drops and increases. How can you tell what is normal everyday variation and which are the prelude to a new epidemic? The choice of algorithm is important as different methods work best in different situations, with different conditions (Buckeridge, 2007).

As you would expect, there are a variety of mathematical techniques to examine this and determine whether what you are seeing is normal, or whether the aberrant points you are currently observing could signal a changing trend. Perhaps the easiest to understand is simply to put in place a threshold. Once cases reach a particular pre-determined level, this signals that a potential outbreak is occurring. When this point is reached an alert is issued or closer investigation can take place. Experience and background knowledge is important in setting a useful threshold here.

However, this is rather imprecise and determining where to place such a threshold somewhat subjective. More common is to use one of a variety of statistical methods. This removes human subjectivity, at least to some extent.

An excellent review article by Faverjon and Berezowski (2018) outline some of the statistical methods available and provides a framework of which to implement in which situation. They divide the methods into what are known as 'statistical process controls' and 'regression'.

Statistical Process Controls
Despite the complex sounding name, this merely means establishing some mean baseline of what is expected, then looking for when the data deviates from this. Another less intimating name that is often used is simply 'control charts'.

A very commonly used method for doing this is the 'Cumulative Summation' method, often shortened to CuSum (O'Brien and Christie, 1997). This basically involves looking at previous historical data points and calculating the mean. Then you can determine whether the current value fits the expected pattern or not. Although ideal in engineering contexts, in epidemiology a problem with this can occur because often the variance in case numbers observed can be high. This means it can often throw out alerts. Refinement using negative binomial distributions can help reduce this. Forms of CuSum has been used in many early syndromic surveillance system, such as the Early Aberration Reporting System (Lawson, 2005).

Other control chart methods include Shewhart charts, which study the difference between observed mean values over a moving time window. More complicated methods such as the use of exponentially weighted moving averages also exist.

Some statistical process control methods for syndromic surveillance

Method
Shewhart charts
Historical limits
EARS
CuSuM
Exponential weighted mean

Regression Analyses
The second major group of methods are those based on regression; essentially you put a line of best fit through your data then look for when cases deviate from this. Regression was described in Chapter 2. A wide variety of methods exist, including the most basic which is linear regression. But there are other more complex techniques which are better suited to disease statistics, including types based on Poisson or negative binomial distributions.

Deciding which method to use takes careful deliberation. Many factors need to be taken into consideration. Which method is best depends on the data which is available, the nature of the condition being examined, and the type of epidemic that might be expected. For example, some forms work best when they have data over a long historical timespan, whereas others are more robust when the amount of data available is minimal. Detailed reviews looking at which method are most suitable in which contexts should be referred to, most widely cited include Unkel et al. (2012), Fricker (2013), and the review referred to earlier by Faverjon and Berezowski (2018).

How widespread is syndromic surveillance?
Although now somewhat dated, the study by Buehler et al. (2003) at least gives an indication of how widely used syndromic surveillance systems are, at least by U.S. public health bodies. In this study the authors surveyed 59 public bodies providing public health provision in the U.S., including the 50 states and additional territories including New York City, Los Angeles, Chicago and the District of Columbia. They received a response from 52 of them.

Of those that responded, 83% said they used syndromic surveillance when questioned 'Do you use any syndromic surveillance systems developed or managed by your health department...?' The most widely used forms involved Emergency Department data (83%), outpatient data (49%), over-the-counter medicine sales data (44%), poison control centre records (37%), and school attendance data (35%). Syndromic surveillance data was examined frequently, with for example emergency department data being looked at daily by 72% of respondents; by 17% more than once a week. Syndromic surveillance was perceived as most effective for spotting large disease outbreaks and influenza, but less so for small outbreak detection.

What the review did not examine was how detailed the form of syndromic surveillance was. Was surveillance 'informal' in nature? Were statistical processes in place for the examination of data, or was only personal judgement used? Given the extent of time that has passed since this study, it is likely that syndromic surveillance is even more widely spread today.

EXAMPLES OF SYNDROMIC SURVEILLANCE SYSTEMS

The National Syndromic Surveillance Program (NSSP)
Organized by the Center for Disease Control (CDC) in the U.S., the National Syndromic Surveillance Program defines what syndromic surveillance is, works to improve outbreak detection, and provides data in an easily accessible manner. For anyone interested in syndromic surveillance this website should be a port of first call because of the range of resources it provides.

Among the dashboards provided in order to help public health professionals understand changes in disease incidence include a tick bite tracker, a COVID-19 dashboard, a heat and health mapper and a drug overdose surveillance system. A monthly newsletter update is also available.

Key to NSSP is the ESSENCE system (Burkom et al. 2021). This is the online program allowing entry of data of importance in syndromic surveillance.

Real-time Syndromic Surveillance Team ReSST

A well documented syndromic surveillance programme is that organised in England by the Health Security Agency (formerly Public Health England). The Real-time Syndromic Surveillance Team (ReSST) collates and interprets data from a wide range of medical sources. The system is described by Morbey et al. (2015). Data used includes both in-hours and out-of-hours GP (general medical practitioner) records (Harcourt et al. 2012), sentinel emergency attendance data (Eliott et al. 2012), and also data from the NHS111 syndromic surveillance system.

Diagnostic codes are used in the examination of records. 'Syndromic indicators', comprised of groups of diagnostic codes, cover a broad range of illnesses of interest for syndromic surveillance including gastrointestinal complaints, and influenza-like-illness. These are collected at a national, regional and local levels (Morbet et al. 2015). Altogether 12,000 signals are recorded each day.

This information is examined using a system of hierarchical mixed effect models, with a separate model being used for each syndromic indicator. These use historical data with regression modelling to assess changes, with historical thresholds being used to identify trends and spot spikes.

Advantages and problems with syndromic surveillance

As already outlined, the main advantage of syndromic surveillance is that is it offers the chance to receive a forewarning of a potential outbreak, allowing preventative measures to be put in place, thus mitigating its impact. Another advantages is price, such systems should be cheap to establish; much of the data is there anyway and just needs to be accessed by the right people, at the right time.

However, there are potential problems which needs to be considered. As mentioned 'false alarms' can occur. Despite having complex statistical procedures in place, these are not foolproof. The issuing of an alert does not necessarily mean there is an epidemic on the way. Also important is whether those producing such alerts are listened to. Having a syndromic surveillance in place is pointless if many reports are written, but no actual pre-emptive action is taken to mitigate potential upcoming problems. For syndromic surveillance to be effective, real action is needed by those responsible for front line health services, not just those in an administrative capacity. Henning (2004) highlighted the need for well defined protocol and administrative procedures to be in place.

The non-specific nature of much syndromic surveillance is a potential problem. It is difficult to infer future case numbers from non-specific symptoms. How many times have you had a sore throat or a cough, but not gone on to develop more serious illness? Katz et al. (2011) identified the fact that symptoms might not relate to the specific illness being examined as a key problem with many studies. A potentially serious outbreak, initially small in number, could easily occur but be masked simply by the sheer number of people experiencing similar symptoms caused by other conditions. Care must be taken not to put too much faith into syndromic surveillance.

Katz et al (2011) also highlighted that additional confusion was caused by many non-syndromic studies calling themselves syndromic, when really they were using data on already diagnosed condition.

Where next?

Syndromic surveillance systems face similar challenges wherever they are. What works well for one symptom group may not work well for another. Determining the best data sources, and the best statistical methods for each context is required. Much future work is thus needed on examining what is best in each situation and then evaluating how effective it is. Therefore, much work is required in tinkering and refining each system to find out what works best in each context. As new methods of analysing data become available, it could well be that better methods of identifying spikes develop and existing systems can be improved.

REFERENCES

Buckeridge DL. Outbreak detection through automated surveillance: A review of the determinants of detection. *Journal of biomedical informatics.* 2007;**40**:370-379.

Buehler JW, Sonricker A, Paladini M, Soper P, Mostashari F. Syndromic surveillance practice in the United States: findings from a survey of state, territorial, and selected local health departments. *Advances in disease surveillance.* 2008;**6**(3):1-20.

Burkom H, Loschen W, Wojcik R, Holtry R, Punjabi M, Siwek M, Lewis S. Electronic surveillance system for the early notification of community-based Epidemics (ESSENCE): Overview, components, and public health applications. *JMIR public health and surveillance.* 2021;**7**(6):e26303.

Elliot AJ, Hughes HE, Hughes TC, Locker TE, Shannon T, Heyworth J, Wapling A, Catchpole M, Ibbotson S, McCloskey B, Smith GE. Establishing an emergency department syndromic surveillance system to support the London 2012 Olympic and Paralympic games. *Emergency medicine journal.* 2012;**29**(12):954-60.

Faverjon C, Berezowski J. Choosing the best algorithm for event detection based on the intended application: a conceptual framework for syndromic surveillance. *Journal of biomedical informatics.* 2018;**85**:126-35.

Fricker RD. Introduction to statistical methods for biosurveillance: with an emphasis on syndromic surveillance. Cambridge University Press; 2013 Feb 25.

Harcourt SE, Smith GE, Elliot AJ, Pebody R, Charlett A, Ibbotson S, Regan M, Hippisley-Cox J. Use of a large general practice syndromic surveillance system to monitor the progress of the influenza A (H1N1) pandemic 2009 in the UK. *Epidemiology and infection.* 2012;**140**(1):100-5.

Henning KJ. What is syndromic surveillance?. *Morbidity and mortality weekly report.* 2004. **24**:7-11.

Lawson BM, Fitzhugh EC, Hall SP, Franklin C, Hutwagner LC, Seeman GM, Craig AS. Multifaceted syndromic surveillance in a public health department using the early aberration reporting system. *Journal of public health management and practice.* 2005;**11**(4):274-81.

Katz R, May L, Baker J, Test E. Redefining syndromic surveillance. *Journal of epidemiology and global health.* 2011;**1**(1):21-31.

Mandl KD, Overhage JM, Wagner MM, Lober WB, Sebastiani P, Mostashari F, Pavlin JA, Gesteland PH, Treadwell T, Koski E, Hutwagner L. Implementing syndromic surveillance: a practical guide informed by the early experience. *Journal of the American medical informatics association.* 2004;**11**(2):141-50.

Morbey RA, Elliot AJ, Charlett A, Verlander NQ, Andrews N, Smith GE. The application of a novel 'rising activity, multi-level mixed effects, indicator emphasis'(RAMMIE) method for syndromic surveillance in England. *Bioinformatics.* 2015;**31**(22):3660-5.

National Institute Clinical Excellence (NICE). Whooping Cough: What else could it be? Clinical Knowledge Summary. 2022. Available at: www.cks.nice.org.uk/topics/whooping-cough/diagnosis/differential-diagnosis/

O'Brien SJ, Christie P. Do CuSums have a role in routine communicable disease surveillance?. *Public health.* 1997;**111**(4):255-8.

Reingold A. If syndromic surveillance is the answer, what is the question? *Biosecurity and bioterrorism.* 2003;**1**:1-5.

World Health Organisation (WHO). Department of Communicable Disease Surveillance and Response. WHO recommended surveillance standards. 2nd ed.; 2001 March 29. Report No. WHO/CDS/CSR/ISR/99.2.

Unkel S, Farrington CP, Garthwaite PH, Robertson C, Andrews N. Statistical methods for the prospective detection of infectious disease outbreaks: a review. *Journal of the royal statistical society: series A (statistics in society).* 2012;**175**(1):49-82.

ACCIDENT AND EMERGENCY ATTENDANCE DATA

Each day we work together as a family because we're a family.

Mark Greene, in the television show ER.

Accident and emergency facilities exist to provide immediate medical treatment for those in urgent need. This could be because someone has had an accident, is taken suddenly seriously unwell, or simply because other healthcare facilities can not be accessed for a variety of reasons. Because of the nature of how these facilities work patients with a great variety of problems often utilize them. Medical staff have little idea who might come through the door next, and what treatments they will require. Thus, an important first step is making an initial assessment and performing triage in order to ensure those most in need of urgent care receive attention first. Following initial assessment patients can be referred as appropriate to receive further care.

Often particularly large hospitals provide walk-in 'ambulatory' healthcare services. Such services are designated for those not seriously ill, but who wish to be seen without appointment immediately. Such services are useful in that they ease pressure on emergency services. An additional advantage is that patients can effectively triage themselves. Our local regional hospital, for example, provides a walk-in eye clinic. If you require treatment for some eye complaint, you simply have to turn up during the opening times and wait to be seen.

Such contact with healthcare services, either through the accident and emergency department or through a walk-in service will result in some record being made. Details of the initial assessment will be recorded, which can be forwarded as and when required. Such information provides a useful potential source for the disease scientist interested in syndromic surveillance.

Treatment, not diagnosis, the priority
It must be borne in mind that the priority for those tasked with dealing with emergency cases is in providing immediate care in order to alleviate pain and suffering. Triage is not diagnosis, just a method of ensuring those in most need are dealt with first. Obviously some form of diagnosis will inevitably occur following contact with medical staff, as unless some idea of the condition being dealt with is known immediate care cannot be best provided.

However, it should be no surprise that occasionally this diagnosis may be incorrect or superficial. This is totally understandable given the time constraints faced by those working in such departments. Detailed diagnosis is often a difficult task, requiring some specialized knowledge and requiring the use of laboratory testing to provide confirmation or rule out alternatives. The symptoms of many conditions are similar. Thus, a fully comprehensive assessment can take several days. The diagnoses made in emergency departments should be seen as educated guesses.

Technology facilitates access to records

As mentioned, once a patient enters an emergency department this will be recorded, along with the initial diagnosis and treatment given. Such information is important to ensure consistency of care and avoid duplication of effort. When referred for further treatment such notes help medical staff along-the-line better understand the patient they have in front of them.

The problem for the epidemiologist is obtaining timely access to such records. Epidemiologists are not one of the chain of healthcare professionals directly involved in providing medical care. Epidemiologists have little interest in the personal details of each specific patient; only in the potential condition they have, when it developed and where. Even if epidemiologists could intercept such information early in the healthcare chain, sifting useful information from the personal clinical information would be a daunting task.

Digital technological developments have greatly changed how such information is stored and communicated. Digital computer based records have replaced traditional paper based ones. This helps ensure accuracy and avoids the mistakes that are inevitable with scribbled notes. It also means information can be passed between people much easier. Crucially, it eases the epidemiologists work in two key ways. Firstly, it means an epidemiologist can access such information totally unobtrusively. Secondly, methods of data retrieval and management mean it is now far easier to filter data to obtain exactly the information that is required to study trends in disease. A public health official sat in a local government office can now gain access to the number of cases of possible influenza admitted each day into hospitals across a wide regional area, without having to leave his or her desk.

Irwin et al. (2003) reported about a surveillance system used in the St. John Hospital, Detroit, MI, which used emergency department data and relied on the process being computerised. At the time of the study the emergency department was receiving 78,000 visits annually. A computer program was written which examined records on a daily basis, and sent an automatic email notifying investigators when the number of patients presenting with specific predefined symptoms was passed.

Large sporting or other events have often been an impetus to the development of syndromic surveillance using accident and emergency data, or at any rate offered the opportunity to assess the effectiveness of such systems. There is concern that the large crowds attending such events, with many visitors coming from abroad, offers the potential for disease outbreaks to start and spread easily. New computerised systems were trialled at the 2012 London Olympics (Elliot et al. 2010) or even at the Kentucky Derby (Carrico et al. 2005).

ICD-10

A key innovation aiding disease monitoring was the development of a standardized method of recording health complaints. Conceived by the World Health Organisation, work on the International Statistical Classification of Diseases and Related Health problems, known universally as ICD, began in 1983. The first completed version became available in 1990 and began to be used by member states from 1994. The currently most widely used version remains ICD-10, although this has recently been superseded by ICD-11 from January 2022.

ICD-10 provides a framework for the standardized classification of health problems. Basically, each recognized condition is assigned a specific and unique code. This ensures that different medical professionals can have some confidence that they are referring to the same condition in discussions with each other. Although studies have shown high correlation between records detailing the chief complaint (Beitel et al. 2004), the use of clinical codes such as ICD codes ensures even greater standardization. It also eases record keeping, meaning there is greater accuracy and it is easier to transfer data. Many countries have interpreted the ICD guidelines to suit their own specific needs, yet retained the general framework provided by the ICD framework. One area where the ICD-10 guidelines have helped epidemiological research is in the use of accident and emergency data, allowing epidemiologists to easily track conditions from the hospital door to referral to subject specialist.

EXAMPLES OF ACCIDENT AND EMERGENCY SURVEILLANCE

An example of accident and emergency surveillance from Taiwan

The study by Wu et al. (2008) is interesting because it found clear spikes in the number of people presenting as emergency cases in certain syndromic categories. Starting in March 2004, data obtained by hospital emergency departments was sent straight to the Taiwanese Center for Disease Control. Examination of this data found clear seasonal peaks in categories for influenza-like-illnesses and other respiratory illness. Although not a surprise, what was interesting was that distinct spikes for certain conditions could be seen. Notably spikes in cases of gastroenteritic conditions were seen which appeared to coincide with school attendance. One potential problem the authors found was that attendance increased during weekends and holiday periods, which could obscure trends.

The Emergency Department Syndromic Surveillance System (EDSSS)

Another example is the Emergency Department Syndromic Surveillance System (EDSSS)(Elliot et al. 2010). This project was established in 2010 in anticipation of the London 2012 Olympic Games. The intention was that it could provide a forewarning of a serious disease outbreak which could be caused by the large numbers of foreign visitors attending the Olympics. The system was a collaboration between the English Health Protection Agency and the College of Emergency Medicine.

The initial study collated key demographic information, triage, and diagnosis codes for those attending accident and emergency departments between July 2010 to 2011 (Elliot et al. 2012). Ultimately this collated data on over 340,000 visits. Visits were categorized into different syndromic groups which included respiratory, gastrointestinal, acute respiratory, cardiac, gastroenteritis, and myocardial ischaemia. Visits for respiratory and acute respiratory reasons peaked in December 2010.

The system was extended and continued as the Real Time Syndromic Surveillance team which was described in Chapter 3 (Hughes et al. 2016). Further study identified seasonal trends in some of the syndromes examined, such as acute respiratory infections.

Biosense and the NSSP

Of especial note is the U.S. Center for Disease Control Biosense system which is part of the National Syndromic Surveillance System for the U.S. (CDC, 2022). This brings together data from a range of settings including emergency departments, outpatient care, and ambulatory care centres onto a single electronic platform which health care professionals can use to assess potential problems and spot early trends. The NSSP website states that over 6,000 care facilities from across the U.S. contribute to Biosense. It thus covers over 70% of emergency visits in the U.S. Data is provided for analysis on a daily basis.

Can such information be used to forecast disease?

These and other studies clearly showed the potential of emergency attendance data. However, most studies simply report the number attending among different syndromic groups. Although such data often shows clear peaks in attendance, for example in specific seasons, few studies actually show whether this data can be used to anticipate trends or spot potential outbreaks any better than conventional surveillance methods. Can such data be used to forecast future levels of disease?

Kim et al. (2019) attempted to do exactly this. The authors examined whether accident and emergency department data could be used to forecast cases of respiratory illness using an ARIMA time series model. They analysed data from Seoul Korea from 2013 to 2015, using the number of patients visiting each day who had elevated temperatures or who were diagnosed with a respiratory illness. Over the two year time period they examined there were over 4 million visits, of which 300,000 were recorded as experiencing symptoms of fever. The authors showed that ARIMA modelling could use such data to forecast future respiratory disease levels. Automatic alarms were triggered when levels role to pre-set warning levels.

Use of emergency attendance data is now widespread

A useful review by Hughes et al. (2020) examined syndromic surveillance systems using emergency data worldwide. It identified 115 systems across 15 countries. The scope of such systems was wide, ranging from local to national, and using a single data source to thousands. National schemes were identified in Albania, France, Jamaica, the Republic of Korea, Singapore and the United Kingdom. The study appeared just as COVID-19 pandemic was in its first year. It will be interesting to see if the COVID-19 pandemic has provided new impetus to the development of new and more integrated systems in the future.

Sentinel medical practitioner records

Sentinel systems based around local medical practitioners are included in this section because these are often the point of first contact for the general public requiring healthcare. In England two systems exist for the monitoring of data from medical practitioners (known in the U.K. as General Practitioners). The General Practise In Hours Syndromic Surveillance (GPIHSS) and General Practise Out of Hours Syndromic Surveillance (GPOOHSS)(Harcourt et al. 2012). These collect diagnostic codes which are then used in the English Syndromic Surveillance system. These developed from an earlier version known as HPA/QSurveillance (Harcourt et al. 2012) which was discontinued in April 2013.

Example studies using accident and emergency data:

Study	Location	Description
Kajita et al. (2017)	Los Angeles, California	Describes a syndromic surveillance system using emergency attendance data centred on the 2015 Special Olympics.
Lober et al. (2003)	King County, Washington State, U.S.	Automatic collation of emergency attendance data based on ICD-9 codes.
Muscatello et al. (2003)	Sydney, Australia	Describes an emergency attendance syndromic surveillance system set up for the 2003 Rugby World Cup.
Thompson et al. (2014)	Winnipeg, Manitoba	Examined whether emergency attendance visits related to influenza. Used data from 'EDIS' which records the chief complaints of those attending. Linear regression analysis showed good fit with lab confirmed cases.

Advantages and disadvantages

An obvious advantage of using emergency department data for disease surveillance is that such data is already being collected. All that is required for such data to be used by epidemiologists are systems to be put into place allowing for the easy retrieval or access to such data. An additional advantage is that such data is collected by qualified and professional healthcare professionals. This means it is likely to be somewhat accurate with the initial diagnoses likely to reflect well the actual condition being suffered.

An important disadvantage is that many patients will only attend such emergency settings when they are already seriously unwell. For influenza-like-illness, for example, it is likely that mild symptoms will develop many days prior to them becoming serious enough to warrant emergency department attendance. Those requiring such medical attention are likely to belong to certain at risk groups, including the elderly or those with pre-existing healthcare conditions. This mean the cases of illness being reported in the emergency setting may well not reflect the general levels of illness present within the general population.

An additional problem is that many of the categories used in the studies mentioned here were rather broad based and generic. Thus, the ability of such surveillance to detect small scale outbreaks of rather specific conditions is questionable. A key impetus in the development of syndromic surveillance systems based on emergency department data was the 2001 anthrax bio-terrorism attack in the U.S. However, it is unlikely that systems based on emergency attendance could spot such anthrax cases. Medical professionals can't be expected to identify rarely occurring conditions with symptoms which mirror more commonly seen ones. Would such a system have detected COVID-19 cases before the symptoms of it were well ascertained?

Where next?

Systems based on emergency department data are likely to become more widespread in the coming decades. Determining which are the best measures to use and methods to implement in order to forecast future spikes or trends is likely to take much research effort.

REFERENCES

Beitel AJ, Olson KL, Reis BY, Mandl KD. Use of emergency department chief complaint and diagnostic codes for identifying respiratory illness in a pediatric population. *Pediatric emergency care.* 2004;**2**(6):355-60.

Carrico, R. Goss, L. Syndromic Surveillance: hospital emergency department participation during the Kentucky Derby festival. *Disaster management and response.* 2005;**3**:73-79.

Center for Disease Control (CDC). National Syndromic Surveillance System. 2022. Available at: www.cdc.gov/nssp/overview.html

Elliot AJ, Hughes HE, Hughes TC, Locker TE, Shannon T, Heyworth J, Wapling A, Catchpole M, Ibbotson S, McCloskey B. Establishing an Emergency Department Syndromic Surveillance System to Support the London 2012 Olympic and Paralympic Games. *Emergency medicine journal.* 2012;**29**:954-960.

Harcourt SE, Smith GE, Elliot AJ, Pebody R, Charlett A, Ibbotson S, Regan M, Hippisley-Cox J. Use of a large general practice syndromic surveillance system to monitor the progress of the influenza A (H1N1) pandemic 2009 in the UK. *Epidemiology and infection.* 2012;**140**(1):100-5.

Hughes HE, Morbey R, Hughes TC, Locker TE, Pebody R, Green HK, Ellis J, Smith GE, Elliot AJ. Emergency department syndromic surveillance providing early warning of seasonal respiratory activity in England. *Epidemiology and infection.* 2016;**144**(5):1052-64.

Hughes HE, Edeghere O, O'Brien SJ, Vivancos R, Elliot AJ. Emergency department syndromic surveillance systems: a systematic review. *BMC public health.* 2020;**20**(1):1-5.

Irvin CB, Nouhan PP, Rice K. Syndromic analysis of computerized emergency department patients' chief complaints: an opportunity for bioterrorism and influenza surveillance. *Annals of emergency medicine.* 2003;**41**:447-52.

Kajita E, Luarca MZ, Wu H, Hwang B, Mascola L. Harnessing syndromic surveillance emergency department data to monitor health impacts during the 2015 Special Olympics World Games. *Public health report.* 2017;**132**:99S-105S.

Kim TH, Hong KJ, Do Shin S, Park GJ, Kim S, Hong N. Forecasting respiratory infectious outbreaks using ED-based syndromic surveillance for febrile ED visits in a Metropolitan City. *The American journal of emergency medicine.* 2019;**37**(2):183-8.

Lober WB, Trigg LJ, Karras BT, Bliss D, Ciliberti J, Duchin JS. Syndromic surveillance using automated collection of computerized discharge diagnosis. *Journal of urban health.* 2003;**80**(Suppl 2):i97-106.

Muscatello DJ, Churches T, Kaldor J, Zheng W, Chiu C, Correll P, Jorm L. An automated, broad-based, near real-time public health surveillance system using presentations to hospital Emergency Departments in New South Wales, Australia. *BMC public health;* 2005;**5**:141.

Thompson LH, Malik MT, Gumel A, Strome T, Mahmud SM. Emergency department and 'Google flu trends' data as syndromic surveillance indicators for seasonal influenza. *Epidemiology and infection.* 2014;**142**(11):2397-405.

Wu TS, Shih FY, Yen MY, Wu JS, Lu SW, Chang KC, Hsiung C, Chou JH, Chu YT, Chang H, Chiu CH. Establishing a nationwide emergency department-based syndromic surveillance system for better public health responses in Taiwan. *BMC public health.* 2008;**8**(1):1-3.

5

CITIZEN SCIENCE

It has been said that democracy is the worst form of
government except all the others that have been tried

Winston Churchill, U.K. premier

Ask people to describe what someone 'doing science' looks like and they will probably provide a description of a man, wearing a white lab coat, who is mixing chemicals in a test tube in a laboratory. Science is a specialist activity, done only by those in formal institutions and formally trained with the relevant qualifications to do so. Science is for professionals; an activity far removed, or at least separate, from everyday society.

However, this image is completely wrong and it always has been. There has always been a place in science for those without formal qualification, not employed by a university or specialist research organization, and the general public. An excellent example is provided by the British Victorian gentlemen scientists of the 19th century; during this time interests such as butterfly collecting, fossil hunting, and even a craze for growing ferns, were popular pastimes. Charles Darwin himself never held an paid academic post as a biologist.

Today, it is possible for everyone to actively participate and contribute to scientific research; whatever there background. Active collaboration with members of the public is a growing area of research for those gathering healthcare data and information about the distribution of disease. Much of this is done using resources such as the internet, email, and digital sensors; so it can be legitimately considered to come under the remit of digital epidemiology. Can public participation help with disease surveillance?

What is citizen science?
Citizen science can be defined as where non-scientifically trained members of the public contribute, collect, collate and potentially even analyse data (Bonney, 2015). Although public participation in science has always occurred, the concept of 'citizen science' itself is a relatively recent phenomenon. A wide variety of citizen science projects exist, being as diverse as people submitting records of bird sightings, to the public actively classifying galaxies (Strasser et al. 2019). At its most simple citizen science can be defined as science conducted by citizens; science by the people (Irwin, 2002).

Literature examining citizen science has blossomed in recent years. Various reviews classify citizen science projects and identify different forms of it. Some classify citizen science depending on the size of the project utilizing it, or its geographical extent (local or national, for example). Often citizen science projects are graded depending on the extent and form in which citizens and non-scientists participate.

Often scientific research is not the main motivation behind a citizen science project, instead it is to engage and connect people with science, the environment and their communities. There are benefits to the participants themselves, who acquire new skills and new knowledge through the process of conducting science (Bonney, 2015). The extent of the educational value gained depends on the project. In some cases citizen science is used as a vehicle to obtain funding, which allows a scientific project to proceed.

Citizen science in the health sciences

Citizen science projects within the health sciences exist, but have mostly concentrated on promoting health education and health literacy rather than being projects where the public actively aid with real research and data collection.

Citizen science is an ideal method with which to promote public health (Minkler et al. 2000). Citizen science can actively engage individuals in the issues affecting their own health, helping them learn about measures they can take to improve their own well being. Much health education involves helping individuals to take responsibility for the decisions that affect their own health and citizen science projects can aid in this. Additionally, such projects can help people to connect with their local communities and learn about health issues at the local level. Classic examples of such projects might include local 'walking for health' groups or local community groups to aid people in stopping smoking.

Although true research projects using the public to help collect research data are rarer, they do exist. Most have examined various environmental factors influencing health, with the public helping in the collection of data. Some excellent examples exist:

- **Measuring air pollution:** A number of studies have used the public to help in the measurement of air pollutants and air quality. For example, Jerrett et al. (2017) fitted members of the public with personal air sensors which recorded the levels of carbon monoxide, nitric oxide, and nitrogen dioxide which participants were exposed to. This method using personal sensors allowed personal differences in exposure to be recorded for the first time. Normally such pollutants are measured using local fixed sensors, which give no indication of individual exposure. The study found a good correlation between personal levels of exposure and government measurements from fixed stations, helping validate the use of personal sensors for such monitoring.

- **Air sensor toolbox:** A project organised by the U.S. Environmental Protection Agency developed an Air Sensor Toolbox for citizen science. Used in Newark, New Jersey, it allowed people to measure particulates in the air themselves, then submit records formally. Individuals could feel they were actively helping with research and felt like true scientists.

- **Atmospheric Aerosols with iSPEX:** Atmospheric aerosols pose a significant health problem, exacerbating a range of conditions including those of the cardiovascular and respiratory systems. However, obtaining data on them is problematic. Information on the size of particulates and their makeup is difficult to obtain over wide geographical areas using automatic testing. Snik et al. (2014) introduced a citizen science project illustrating how people can be integrated into the measuring regime. They distributed a smartphone add on, called the iSPEX, which allowed users to measure atmospheric aerosols. Users had to actively orientate the device correctly and take repeated measurements in a correct manner.

The Dutch based study involved the distribution of 8,000 iSPEX devices and a national measuring day, which resulted in over 6,000 measurements being obtained across the entire country. Additional testing days resulted in over a thousand additional records on each day. The study was able to study atmospheric quality across time for an entire country, providing a quantity of data which a small group of researches working alone would not have been able to obtain.

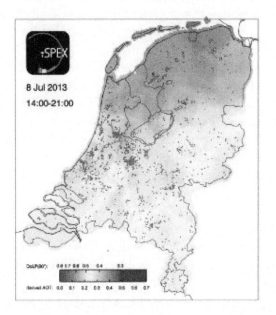 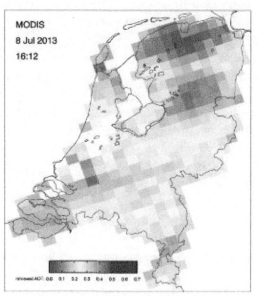

Image from the iSPEX website showing, left, results from public submission of data on air quality, and right, data from a remote satellite for comparison. Map is for July 8, 2013. Dots indicate individual data submissions (there were over 6,000). The underlying colour/shading indicates air quality, which is produced using an average of local submissions. Available from: www.ispex.nl/en

Disease surveillance

Although a number of platforms exist for the public to help with disease surveillance, few studies have stated that they are 'citizen science' projects. Public participation is particularly suitable for the study of vector borne diseases. Thus it is not the disease itself that is being monitored, but the principal vector instead. One example is provided by a Canadian long term study where citizen participants were involved in tick surveillance. Volunteers proved as effective as 'academic' tick collectors. A small number of volunteers were particularly active and dedicated. The data collected by these citizen scientists was used to help understand trends in associated Lyme disease (Lewis et al. 2018).

Mosquito Alert was started in 2014 and is a citizen science platform allowing participants to submit sightings of mosquitoes (Palmer et al. 2017; Tyson et al. 2018). Originally focused on Spain and the mosquito species *Aedes albopictus*, it now has worldwide coverage and covers a variety of species including *Aedes aegyptii* and species of the *Culex* genus. Participants use their smartphones to report adult mosquito sightings, with photos being validated by scientists. It has proved most successful, with more than 821,000 reports being made from 33,000 people (Carney et al. 2022). An example of its utility was shown when it was able to track the progression of *Aedes albopictus* in Spain as this species moved into new areas (Eritja et al. 2019).

Another example is provided by GLOBE, Global Learning and Observations to Benefit the Environment. This is a platform allowing the public participation in monitoring environmental parameters (Low, 2021). One section concentrates on mosquito monitoring and contains the Mosquito Habitat Mapper. This allows participants to submit photos of both adult and larval mosquitoes. An important feature is that it prompts participants to eliminate the open water source where mosquitoes were observed, thus combining both disease surveillance with health education and helping reduce mosquito borne disease directly (Gu et al. 2006).

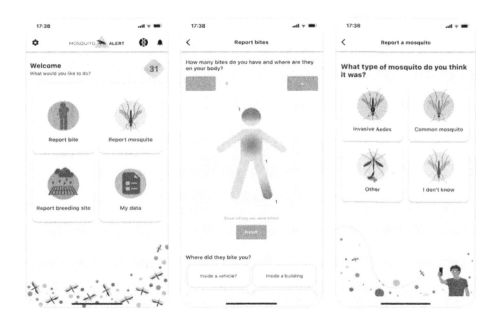

Mosquito Alert by John Palmer is a mobile phone app allowing members of the public to record mosquito sightings.

PatientsLikeMe

The internet has allowed people to connect and interact with each other in ways that were not imaginable previously. In 1998 builder and architect Stephen Heywood was diagnosed with a form of Motor Neurone Disease known as Lou Gehrig's disease. What would happen? Which treatments would work? What had other patients with this condition experienced previously? Stephen wanted to know from others affected by this condition, but could not contact them.

The internet provided a method of communication with others who had been similarly affected. In 2006 Stephen set up a website 'PatientsLikeMe', for those with the same condition as himself so that they could share experiences and information. It soon expanded to cover other conditions such as Parkinson's disease and HIV/AIDS. From 2011 it was available for people with any condition. PatientsLikeMe is more than simply a website. It allows users to record treatments and disease progression, and access the latest research and developments.

Aiding research and finding ways to improve treatment were key motivations behind the development of PatientsLikeMe (Wicks, et al. 2010). An example in how it has helped this is provided by where patient experiences helped in the development of a scoring system for multiple sclerosis (Wicks et al. 2011). However, it must be borne in mind that PatientsLikeMe is a private company working closely with pharmaceutical companies such as Genetech and Novartis. This poses some potential dilemmas; such companies are motivated by profits. Who owns information submitted by the public? And who decides how it will be used?

COVID-19 and the ZOE Symptom Tracker

In the broadest sense, mobile apps reliant on public participation can be considered a form of citizen science. Research utilising such technology and dependant on public participation became prominent during the COVID-19 pandemic.

The COVID-19 Symptom Tracker was used early in the COVID-19 pandemic to study potential symptoms (Drew et al. 2020). It was developed by the research company ZOE International, along with researchers at King's College, London and Massachusetts General Hospital in the U.S. Later renamed the ZOE Health Study, it was based upon a mobile phone app. People, whether they believed they had COVID-19 or not, were urged to download the app and report basic information about themselves and whether they experienced any symptoms.

In the Spring of 2020 little was known about COVID-19. Although it was known to be a severe respiratory illness it was uncertain what the initial symptoms were. Did those contracting the virus develop any characteristic symptoms which because they appeared minor were being missed by researchers? What about those who did not go on to develop severe illness? Were the symptoms they developed different from those developing serious illness? Could the number of people contracting the infection be estimated from the numbers reporting symptoms? The Symptom Tracker aimed to answer these questions.

In March 2020, the app was quickly rolled out in the U.K. On its initial release over a million people downloaded it. An article in May 2020 reported that there were 2.4 million users in the U.K. with 789,000 reporting they had symptoms (Menni et al. 2020). Of the 15,000 participants who had been tested for COVID-19 6,400 proved to be positive, with 64% of these reporting a loss of smell and taste as a symptom. The study found that other symptoms associated with infection included fever, persistent cough, fatigue, shortness of breath, diarrhoea, delirium, skipped meals, abdominal pain, chest pain and a hoarse voice. Using the data they were able to predict that 17% of those experiencing compatible symptoms were likely to have had COVID-19. Interestingly, they also found an effect of media coverage. After the media reported that loss of smell and taste were potential symptoms, these began being reported more by participants from the U.K.

The potential of 'wearables'
Over the past decade personal devices to monitor personal health status, collectively referred to as 'wearables', have become commonplace. They include products such as the FitBit or Apple Watch. Such devices offer much promise to improve personal health care and to help epidemiology (Munos et al. 2016). The idea is to collect data about yourself meaning you can better understand your own health, and potentially provide information to the doctors and clinicians who might need to treat you. In effect you are doing 'personal science' on yourself. An advantage of such devices is that they offer people the chance to learn about there own body and develop personal expertise about healthcare (Heyen, 2020).

Can data from such wearables be used for public health research purposes? Interest increased during the COVID-19 pandemic. It was realized that wearables can potentially monitor symptoms, some of which may indicate infectious disease. It should be feasible for such individual information to be collected then collated centrally to track centres of possible disease outbreak. It could be possible, for example, to track COVID-19 on the basis of individual symptoms (Sen-Crowe, 2020). Monitoring for symptoms such as fever (Smarr et al. 2020) and influenza (Tzovaras, 2021) has been shown to be feasible.

The U.K. Biobank
The U.K. Biobank was established in the early 2000's as a resource where information about a large number of people is available, all of whom are willing to help scientific research. As such it can be considered a citizen science project of sorts. It is ideal to investigate topics such as the factors influencing long term conditions such as diabetes and heart disease. It provides a unique resource for researchers needing access to large sample sizes of participants. 500,000 people between the ages of 40 and 69 signed up between 2006 and 2010. Participants provide basic data relating to their age, gender, and socioeconomic background (Ollier et al. 2005; Sudlow et al. 2015). Data is de-identified and then made available to researchers. Should researchers need to find people willing to provide more information or to actively participate in research they can be contacted. Examples of this include participants being contacted on order to complete web based questionnaires.

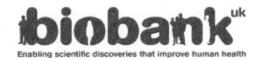

Our Future Health

Already in the process of being established is the Our Future Health (2022) project in the U.K. This aims to collect and collate data from initially three million people, with the hope of eventually being open to everyone in the U.K. Invitations to potential participants began being sent out in the Autumn of 2022, initially to adults in London, West Yorkshire, the West Midlands and Greater Manchester. Participants were asked to fill in detailed questionnaires, provide blood samples and potentially take genetic tests. The project is a collaboration between the British National Health Service and a number of charities including the British Heart Foundation and Diabetes U.K. Also collaborating are a number of industry partners including AstraZeneca. The ultimate aim is to enable population wide research into health problems and diseases.

Advantages of citizen science

The obvious advantage of citizen science projects are that they enable research to be conducted at a scale that simply can't be managed by either a single researcher or a small research team. Far greater amounts of data and information can be collected by engaging thousands, potentially millions, of willing helpers. Not only is the potential quantity of data that can be collected far greater than what lone researchers can obtain, but it also typically comes from a wider geographical area and a wider diversity of people.

Typically, the people we meet on a daily basis are just like us; in background, heritage, and socio-economic status. And this applies to researchers and the people they typically use in research studies as well. Citizen science projects can break down these barriers allowing data on a far wider range of people to be collected. By doing so citizen science can increase the knowledge base of which research is made up from (Irwin, 2002). This benefit of this should not be underestimated. Local knowledge, or personal experiences, can enhance thinking. Contextual knowledge is often essential for effective data interpretation, and cooperation with people actually affected by health conditions can help researchers gain such understanding.

Citizen science increases public interest and engagement in science (Haywood et al. 2013). For those participating in citizen science projects in the health sciences this has particular benefits. For example, it is easy to see how a person contributing to a citizen science project about diet and weight might actively go on to change their own dietary habits, or seek out information to help them do so. Once people have contributed to a project they are more likely to feel ownership and thus responsibility for it. People are more likely to trust knowledge that they themselves have contributed to.

Disadvantages of citizen science

A question that often occurs with data collected via citizen science projects is that of quality. How accurate is the data being collected? How reliable are those submitting it? A useful example is to consider data collected through an online survey where participants answer a series of questions about their health. How truthful are participants being when answering such questions? Maybe they provide the answers that they think researchers want. Maybe this is not even done consciously. If you were asked how many cream buns you had last week, would you be honest, even to yourself?

Citizen science projects experience similar problems which occur with other forms of surveying, such as sampling bias. Those willing to engage in citizen science projects are likely to have more outgoing, open personalities than maybe is the norm. For example, it is easy to imagine that a citizen science project studying cycling and health attracts those already actively exercising on a regular basis. Those taking part in citizen science projects may potentially act differently and have different health needs than those who do not take part in such projects.

Are citizen science projects really 'true' scientific research? Steiner et al. (2020) provides an example of a citizen science project where members of the public studied local mosses to determine the levels of pollution being emitted from a local steel recycling plant. But the authorities did not later use the data collected. This sent a powerful message to the community that evidence can be ignored by the authorities if does not fit what is expected or wanted. Taking part in citizen science projects can be incredibly rewarding for those involved, but where the knowledge is collected then not used this can be incredibly demotivating.

Den Broeder (2018) provides an anecdote of a council led citizen science project run to engage a community close to the Dutch city of Amsterdam with weight control. The project had to be abandoned as this objective did not meet the concerns of the community involved. Citizen science only works if the community are interested in the project and see some relevance in it to themselves.

Are citizens really participating in citizen science?
When is a research project really a citizen science project and when not? When are the public participating and when simply being monitored? As technology progresses the level of participation required is becoming often increasingly minimal. When is the point reached that projects are no longer really participatory. For example, can people really be said to be participating in a health research project if at the end of the day all the data is being collected automatically, and all participants have to do is consent that it be sent to a remote researcher?

The trend for increasing automation is occurring across science generally. Once data collection was often the principle activity of researchers, taking up significant amounts of their time. But increasingly researchers now do not actually play any part in data collection themselves, simply accessing it from a server or portal. Thus although people may wish to engage with scientists through citizen science projects, the researchers if anything can be even more remote.

In some respects many of the studies mentioned in following parts of this book could also be considered as being citizen science projects. After all, any study examining health of individuals requires some participation by the people included in the study. In this chapter I have concentrated on providing examples where people played a more active part in data collection; and had to decide what to submit and whether to submit it themselves.

Examples of national mosquito tracking programs. Members of the public submit sightings to help track vector borne disease.

Program	Country
iMoustique)	France
Mückenatlas	Germany
Muggenradar	Netherlands
Mosquito Reporting Scheme and Mosquito Watch	U.K.
Mosquito Stoppers	U.S.A.

Where next?

Unlike the other chapters in this book which mainly cover discrete and single resources that can be used to source useful data from, citizen science is more a concept. It encompasses a wide range of methods of engaging the public themselves in data collection and even analysis. Of all the methods outlined in this book, citizen science arguably offers the greatest future potential. If anything it is up to the researchers themselves to initiate projects and reach out to communities, make connections, and develop the links that will allow people to engage with research. New technological inventions, such as 'wearables', can only make this an even more fruitful and worthy field of investigation.

REFERENCES

Bonney R, Phillips TB, Ballard HL, Enck JW. Can citizen science enhance public understanding of science? *Public understanding of science*. 2015;**25**(1):2-16.

Carney RM, Mapes C, Low RD, Long A, Bowser A, Durieux D, Rivera K, Dekramanjian B, Bartumeus F, Guerrero D, Seltzer CE. Integrating global citizen science platforms to enable next-generation surveillance of invasive and vector mosquitoes. *Insects*. 2022;**13**(8):675.

Den Broeder L, Devilee J, Van Oers H, Schuit AJ, Wagemakers A. Citizen science for public health. *Health promotion international*. 2018;**33**(3):505-14.

Drew DA, Nguyen LH, Steves CJ, Menni C, Freydin M, Varsavsky T, Sudre CH, Cardoso MJ, Ourselin S, Wolf J, Spector TD. Rapid implementation of mobile technology for real-time epidemiology of COVID-19. *Science*. 2020;**368**(6497):1362-7.

Eritja R, Ruiz-Arrondo I, Delacour-Estrella S, Schaffner F, Álvarez-Chachero J, Bengoa M, Puig MÁ, Melero-Alcíbar R, Oltra A, Bartumeus F. First detection of *Aedes japonicus* in Spain: An unexpected finding triggered by citizen science. *Parasites and vectors*. 2019;**12**:53.

Gu W, Regens JL, Beier JC, Novak RJ. Source reduction of mosquito larval habitats has unexpected consequences on malaria transmission. *Proceedings of the national academy of sciences*. 2006;**103**(46):17560-3.

Haywood BK, Parrish JK, Dolliver J. Place-based and data-rich citizen science as a precursor for conservation action. *Conservation biology*. 2016;**30**(3):476-86.

Heyen NB. From self-tracking to self-expertise: the production of self-related knowledge by doing personal science. *Public understanding of science.* 2020;**29**(2):124-138

Irwin A. Citizen science: A study of people, expertise and sustainable development. Routledge; 2002.

Jerrett M, Donaire-Gonzalez D, Popoola O, Jones R, Cohen RC, Almanza E, De Nazelle A, Mead I, Carrasco-Turigas G, Cole-Hunter T, Triguero-Mas M. Validating novel air pollution sensors to improve exposure estimates for epidemiological analyses and citizen science. *Environmental research.* 2017;**158**:286-94.

Lewis J, Boudreau CR, Patterson JW, Bradet-Legris J, Lloyd VK. Citizen science and community engagement in tick surveillance—a Canadian case study. *Healthcare* 2018;6:22.

Low RD, Schwerin TA, Boger R, Soeffing C, Nelson PV, Bartlett D, Kimura M, Ingle P, Clark A. Building international capacity for citizen scientist engagement in mosquito surveillance and mitigation: The GLOBE Program's GLOBE Observer Mosquito Habitat Mapper. *Insects.* 2022;**13**:624.

Low R, Boger R, Nelson P, Kimura M. GLOBE Mosquito Habitat Mapper citizen science data 2017–2020. *Geohealth.* 2021;**5**(10):e2021GH000436.

Menni C, Valdes AM, Freidin MB, Sudre CH, Nguyen LH, Drew DA, Ganesh S, Varsavsky T, Cardoso MJ, El-Sayed Moustafa JS, Visconti A. Real-time tracking of self-reported symptoms to predict potential COVID-19. *Nature medicine.* 2020;**26**(7):1037-40.

Minkler M. Using participatory action research to build healthy communities. *Public health reports.* 2000;**115**(2-3):191.

Munos B, Baker PC, Bot BM, Crouthamel M, de Vries G, Ferguson I, Hixson JD, Malek LA, Mastrototaro JJ, Misra V, Ozcan A. Mobile health: the power of wearables, sensors, and apps to transform clinical trials. *Annals of the New York academy of sciences.* 2016;**1375**(1):3-18.

Ollier W, Sprosen T, Peakman T. UK Biobank: from concept to reality.

Our Future Health. Project Website. 2022. Available at: www //ourfuturehealth.org.uk

Palmer JR, Oltra A, Collantes F, Delgado JA, Lucientes J, Delacour S, Bengoa M, Eritja R, Bartumeus F. Citizen science provides a reliable and scalable tool to track disease-carrying mosquitoes. *Nature communications.* 2017;**8**(1):1-3.

Sen-Crowe B, McKenney M, Elkbuli A. Utilizing technology as a method of contact tracing and surveillance to minimize the risk of contracting COVID-19 infection. *American journal of emerging medicine.* 2021;**45**:519

Smarr BL, Aschbacher K, Fisher SM, Chowdhary A, Dilchert S, Puldon K, Rao A, Hecht FM, Mason AE. Feasibility of continuous fever monitoring using wearable devices. *Scientific reports.* 2020;**10**(1):1-1.

Snik F, Rietjens JH, Apituley A, Volten H, Mijling B, Di Noia A, Heikamp S, Heinsbroek RC, Hasekamp OP, Smit JM, Vonk J. Mapping atmospheric aerosols with a citizen science network of smartphone spectropolarimeters. *Geophysical research letters.* 2014;**41**(20):7351-8.

Steiner SM. Popular epidemiology and community-based citizen science: using a bio-indicator for toxic air pollution. SAGE Publications Ltd; 2020.

Strasser B, Baudry J, Mahr D, Sanchez G, Tancoigne E. " Citizen science"? Rethinking science and public participation. *Science and technology studies.* 2019;**32**:52-76.

Sudlow C, Gallacher J, Allen N, Beral V, Burton P, Danesh J, Downey P, Elliott P, Green J, Landray M, Liu B. UK biobank: an open access resource for identifying the causes of a wide range of complex diseases of middle and old age. *Plos medicine.* 2015;**12**(3):e1001779.

Tyson E, Bowser A, Palmer J, Kapan D, Bartumeus F, Brocklehurst M, Pauwels E. Global Mosquito Alert. Woodrow Wilson International Center for Scholars, Washington, DC. 2018. Available at: wilsoncenter.org/publication/global-mosquito-alert-building-citizen-science-capacity-for-surveillance-and-control

Tzovaras BG, Hidalgo ES, Alexiou K, Baldy L, Morane B, Bussod I, Fribourg M, Wac K, Wolf G, Ball M. Using an individual-centered approach to gain insights from wearable data in the quantified flu platform: netnography study. *Journal of medical internet research.* 2021;**23**(9):e28116.

Wicks P, Massagli M, Frost J, Brownstein C, Okun S, Vaughan T, Bradley R, Heywood J. Sharing health data for better outcomes on PatientsLikeMe. *Journal of medical internet research.* 2010;**12**(2):e1549.

Wicks P, Massagli M, Kulkarni A, Dastani H. Use of an online community to develop patient-reported outcome instruments: the Multiple Sclerosis Treatment Adherence Questionnaire (MS-TAQ). *Journal of medical internet research.* 2011;**13**(1):e1687.

HELPLINE AND EMERGENCY CALL DATA

What's your emergency?

**Title of a British television
documentary running from 2012.**

Telephone contact with healthcare services can be made for a number of reasons. Often what Springs to mind first is the emergency phone 999 service here in the U.K., or 911 in the U.S. However, far more common are telephone calls made by people wanting to book routine appointments with medical surgeries or outpatient departments. Such telephone calls are increasingly being managed through centralized call centres. There is also an increasing trend for healthcare providers to provide telephone helplines to act as a point of first contact, providing an initial source of help and advice. Such services aim to make healthcare services as accessible as possible and also hopefully relieve pressure on physical healthcare services. With the advent of the COVID-19 pandemic, medical consultations themselves routinely began to take place remotely, usually via telephone or through internet video calls, with face-to-face contact only occurring where strictly necessary.

Such telephone calls offer another potential data source for those studying trends in disease and wanting to spot disease outbreaks. Records of calls made through centralized telephone systems are typically logged automatically. Has such data been used in epidemiology?

Telephone triage

It can be difficult to gain an accurate assessment of a callers needs and requirements over the telephone. The only information a telephonist has is what the caller tells them. Which questions are the best to find the information the telephonist requires? Additionally, such medical and healthcare telephone services can experience high volumes of calls. It makes sense to prioritise those calls requiring immediate attention. The telephone operator has the job of performing such assessment and re-directing callers onwards to the appropriate service.

Thus, telephone triage is necessary, with some initial assessment of calls typically occurring as they are made in order to better manage services. Often a well defined protocol is followed, with callers being asked certain specific questions aimed at best meeting their needs and providing the telephonist with the information required as quickly as possible.

Early studies examining telephone data

Considerable research has gone into assessing whether such telephone triage data can be used to provide an early indication of potential healthcare issues, disease outbreaks and overall trends. One of the earliest to examine this was the research outlined in Rodman (1998), which showed that there was a 17-fold increase in calls about diarrhoea to a nursing hotline in Millwaukee, Wisconsin following an outbreak of cryptosporidiosis in 1993. Seasonal trends for conditions such as diarrhoea and vomiting were apparent, with the number of calls peaking in Winter months when these conditions were most prevalent.

Another early example using telephone health data comes from the Ontario Telehealth System, known usually in its shortened form simply as 'telehealth'. This system is described in the work of Rolland et al. (2006). The system started in 2001 and provides telephone health support to residents of Ontario 24 hours a day. At the time of the 2006 study it was receiving 3,000 calls daily, with registered nurses providing advice. In a prospective study the baseline threshold number of calls on conditions was ascertained for key symptom groups such as gastrointestinal, constitutional, respiratory, rash, haemorrhagic, botulinic, neurological, and other. This provided a basis for comparison in later studies. The system was later used by Caudle et al. (2009) who examined gastrointestinal complaints and showed that calls to telehealth about these complaints showed a strong correlation to corresponding national emergency discharge data.

Inevitably, because of the burden it places on healthcare services, much emphasis has been on whether telephone and call centre data can spot peaks in influenza before they can be spotted through other methods. One of the earliest studies examining the use of telephone call data to examine influenza was by Espino et al. (2003). This study examined call centre data from a group of hospital emergency room triage centres and a centralized after hours telephone service for a group of state medical practitioners. The study used data for the influenza year 2001 to 2002, with the authors using the coding on calls to assess which were influenza related. They then compared this data with national CDC datasets for influenza to examine whether trends in telephone calls occurred prior to official recorded case numbers and emergency data. The data for emergency room telephone triaging was able to determine a peak in influenza earlier than CDC official sources, although this did not occur for the corresponding data for medical practitioner telephone triage data.

NHS Direct and NHS111

A good example of how calls can be processed is provided by U.K.'s telephone NHS111 service. This was first established as 'NHS Direct' in 2011. This was meant to provide a point of first contact for those with health issues and concerns, and by offering an easy method of contact aimed to ease the burden on overstretched medical surgeries and hospital accident and emergency departments. It also aimed to increase accessibility to NHS services for those groups where barriers existed to obtaining NHS care. From 2014 NHS Direct became NHS111, integrating both telephone and internet services into one in order to provide a more joined up service. Data on the number of calls received by NHS111 is made publicly available (Nuffield Trust, 2022).

What happens when you ring NHS111? A computer program which contains various algorithms prompts the telephonist to ask a series of questions. This is known as NHS Pathways. The sequence of questions asked depends on the answers provided to each prior question. The algorithms use the answers provided to classify cases and prompt the telephonist to provide the appropriate information. These algorithms thus help the most urgent cases to be given priority. Calls are classified into symptom types as part of this system; such classification is ideal for syndromic surveillance.

Weekly reports for syndromic surveillance

Details of calls are logged which provides data which can later be analysed by epidemiologists. A 'Public Health England Real-time Syndromic Surveillance Team' was established soon after NHS Digital started. It now uses data from the NHS111 service to produce weekly reports (U.K. Health Security Agency, 2022). Originally this team used data from what was then known as the 'CAS' system, which has now been superseded by the Pathways system (NHS, 2022). A control chart system is used, with data being compared over comparable previous time units. This means unusual rises in syndromes, such as vomiting, can be spotted (Baker et al. 2003).

As part of this project, the UK Health Security Agency produces weekly reports on trends in symptoms using data obtained from the NHS111 system, and also using data obtained directly from medical surgeries. Commonplace symptoms such as coughs, fever, and vomiting, indicative of a wide range of potential conditions, are recorded. Weekly reports on trends for these key symptoms are produced showing the rates of symptoms per 100,000 and providing a breakdown by age range. These reports are quite extensive and produced on a regular interval, meaning that trends can hopefully be spotted.

NHS Direct and influenza

Harcourt et al. (2001) identified the potential such telephone data could offer in tracking levels of influenza in a pilot study using NHS Direct data. Although this study used data from only one influenza season, 1999, the viability of using such data for syndromic surveillance was demonstrated. A follow-up study using data from later years was performed (Cooper et al. 2002).

Another notable study is that of Cooper et al. (2009) which looked at NHS Direct data relating to the 'cold/flu' and 'fever' categories in CAS data. This examined the number of calls received under the 'cold/flu' category for all ages, and those for 'fever' for those under five and between 5 to 14 years of age. Using Poisson distribution modelling the numbers were compared to those recorded as having influenza-like-illness from sentinel doctor surgeries data from the Royal College of General Practice (RCGP). The authors determined that when a threshold of 1.2% of calls related to fever (using data from all age categories) was passed, or 9% of calls for fever in the 5 to 14 age ranges, then this provided a two week warning of when an influenza peak was likely to occur.

Work by Morbey et al. (2017) examined calls made to NHS111 between 2013 and 2015 and looked at the relationship between calls and laboratory confirmed and recorded respiratory illnesses during this period. There was a strong association between telephone calls on coughs, colds and difficulties breathing with laboratory recorded cases of Respiratory Syncytial Virus (RSV) and influenza. Calls about coughing in young children were particularly strongly associated with RSV levels. Modelling showed that using call volume data could anticipate corresponding changes in the laboratory test data by one week.

Norovirus and NHS calls

Infection with norovirus causes vomiting sickness which can last several days (Robilotti et al. 2015). This is merely a highly unpleasant illness to those who are relatively healthy. However, for those in an already weakened state it can be much more serious, resulting in a range of health complications and exacerbating other health conditions.

Annual peaks in norovirus cases occur, typically during the Winter months. Outbreaks are often centred on hospital settings. Being able to predict when exactly these peaks will be most likely to occur would be most useful, especially for those tasked with caring for vulnerable or elderly patients who could take appropriate preventative measures. However, traditional surveillance based upon examining the results from routine laboratory testing often does not provide a timely enough signal for when such peaks will occur. Could calls to the NHS111 service provide an earlier indication?

Loveridge et al (2010) looked at whether peaks in the numbers of hospital based norovirus cases could be anticipated by examining calls to the NHS Direct/NHS111 system. The authors examined the proportion of calls for gastroenteritis (non-rotavirus) and vomiting. They found that when the proportion of calls for these symptoms reached 4% over a two week period, this provided about four weeks advanced notice of an impending peak in norovirus.

Gastroenteritis and Swedish Health Care Direct 1177

Another study by Andersson et al. (2014) compared different syndromic surveillance systems and there ability to pick up outbreaks of gastrointestinal illness. The authors gathered data from the Swedish telephone health service 'Swedish Health Care Direct' 1177. This records the reason for a contact call, and notes the main symptom experienced by the callers. The researchers looked at records for gastrointestinal illness which covered five main symptoms.

They also gathered data from the Swedish Vardguiden website which offers health advice in Swedish. And finally they obtained data about 'over-the-counter' sales of medication that could be purchased to relieve symptoms of gastrointestinal illness. Over the time period examined, 2007 to 2011, there were nine gastrointestinal disease outbreaks. Three of these were caused by contaminated water and three by contaminated food. The researchers examined the four largest outbreaks and found that all four could be spotted using the 1177 telephone data. Only two could be spotted using the 'over-the-counter' sales data. Whilst none could be identified using the data from internet search records. Importantly, the peaks in telephone call data occurred notably earlier than peaks in actual case numbers, thus showing that this data could provide a useful forewarning. Increases in sales data occurred two to four days slower than corresponding increases in telephone calls.

COVID-19 and coronavirus triage

During the COVID-19 pandemic those contacting the NHS through either the NHS111 telephone helpline system, 111 online, or the emergency 999 number, were assessed for COVID-19 symptoms. If such symptoms were identified then the callers could be provided with appropriate advice and signposted as to where to obtain further guidance.

Data on the numbers of assessments made was recorded, along with information on the geographical location and personal characteristics of the callers. This data was collated nationally, with results being published at regular intervals on a specialist website.

This was arguably one of the best uses of telephone triage data in the U.K. to date. It allowed the effective mapping of areas of the U.K. where COVID-19 levels could be rising. From the 18th of March 2020 to July 2022 a total of 2,686,946 triages for COVID-19 occurred (NHS Digital, 2022).

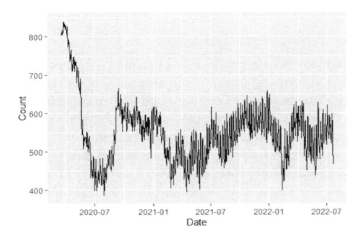

The number of calls made to NHS111 during the COVID-19 pandemic. Note the large drop from the peak in early 2020, and seasonal variations. Data from NHS Digital (2022).

Advantages and disadvantages

A big advantage of data obtained from telephone health lines is there immediacy. Using telephone triage data offers a chance to gather information about potential outbreaks before a patient even sees a clinician and a diagnosis is made. Information is gathered about potential cases before severe illness develops. Information is obtained about those in the first stages of illness who feel unwell and simply require advice and guidance. Most people are reluctant to attend medical practitioners before they are really unwell, most attempting to self treat in the initial phases of illness. Typically, appointments are only made to see a medical practitioner only once someone is seriously unwell.

This is perfect for epidemiologists who want to obtain any indication of potential outbreaks or peaks in infection as early as possible. Although this might mean some of the cases recorded are 'false alarms', given a large enough volume of calls, true trends will become apparent. Although potentially not as accurate as a diagnosis performed by clinical staff and backed up with laboratory testing, the telephonists are often trained in patient assessment, and the use of guiding software with appropriate questions, means data of a reliable enough standard can be obtained for disease surveillance purposes.

Other advantages include that obtaining such data should be relatively easy; records on the telephone calls received through such services are made anyway. All that is needed is a system allowing such data to be forwarded to an appropriate professional so that it can be analysed. Today, such processes can be automated with alerts being issued if the number of calls on specific symptoms passes some pre-set threshold.

However, there are some disadvantages to the use of telephone call data. Typically such systems will be best for the surveillance of relatively common conditions. The large number of calls received for common conditions will mean that incorrect diagnosis and other 'noise' in the data will be less important. The general underlying trends will be clearer. However, there is less chance that such a system will identify outbreaks of relatively rare conditions or clusters of cases occurring in a localised area. Rare conditions may not be looked for, and are easily missed especially by those used to seeing a large number of commoner conditions. As with other syndromic surveillance systems, the problem of conditions sharing multiple symptoms can be problematic. Data on a single symptom in isolation is unlikely to be of much use.

Where next?

Data obtained from telephone helplines has long been recognized as a potential source of information for those interested in disease outbreak detection. However, it is only really in the last decade that organised systems for its systematic analysis have been developed and implemented by national health organisations. The development of new analysis techniques such as time frequency analysis means that it is becoming easier to spot anomalies in time series maybe indicative of developing outbreaks. An important next step is determining exactly which form of analysis is best suited to each specific context. As more data showing the effectiveness of such data over longer periods of time is obtained, systems can be refined and improved and the best markers and indicators of potential outbreaks identified. Further research needs to examine which symptoms are associated with which conditions and how effective examination of these is for determining peaks in incidence of specific conditions before they occur.

REFERENCES

Andersson T, Bjelkmar P, Hulth A, Lindh J, Stenmark S, Widerström M. Syndromic surveillance for local outbreak detection and awareness: evaluating outbreak signals of acute gastroenteritis in telephone triage, web-based queries and over-the-counter pharmacy sales. *Epidemiology and infection.* 2014;**142**(2):303-13.

Baker M, Smith GE, Cooper D, Verlander NQ, Chinemana F, Cotterill S, Hollyoak V, Griffiths R. Early warning and NHS Direct: a role in community surveillance? *Journal of public health medicine.* 2003;**25**:362-8.

Caudle JM, van Dijk A, Rolland E, Moore KM. Telehealth Ontario detection of gastrointestinal illness outbreaks. *Canadian journal of public health.* 2009;**100**(4):253-7.

Cooper DL, Verlander NQ, Elliot AJ, Joseph CA, Smith GE. Can syndromic thresholds provide early warning of national influenza outbreaks?. *Journal of public health.* 2009;**31**(1):17-25.

Cooper DL, Smith GE, Hollyoak VA, Joseph CA, Johnson L, Chaloner R. Use of NHS Direct calls for surveillance of influenza – a second year's experience. *Communicable disease and public health.* 2002;**5**:127-31.

Espino JU, Hogan WR, Wagner MM. Telephone triage: a timely data source for surveillance of influenza-like diseases. In: AMIA Annual Symposium Proceedings 2003 (Vol. 2003, p. 215). American Medical Informatics Association.

Harcourt SE, Smith GE, Hollyoak V, Joseph CA, Chaloner R, Rehman Y, Warburton F, Ejidokun OO, Watson JM, Griffiths RK. Can calls to NHS Direct be used for syndromic surveillance? *Communicable disease and public health.* 2001;**4**:178-82.

Loveridge P, Cooper D, Elliot AJ, Harris J, Gray J, Large S, Regan M, Smith GE, Lopman B. Vomiting calls to NHS Direct provide an early warning of norovirus outbreaks in hospitals. *Journal of hospital infection.* 2010;**74**(4):385-93.

Morbey RA, Harcourt S, Pebody R, Zambon M, Hutchison J, Rutter J, Thomas H, Smith GE, Elliot AJ. The burden of seasonal respiratory infections on a national telehealth service in England. *Epidemiology and infection.* 2017;**145**(9):1922-32.

National Health Service (NHS). Pathways. 2022. Available at: https://digital.nhs.uk/dashboards/nhs-pathways

NHS Digital. Potential Coronavirus (COVID-19) symptoms reported through NHS Pathways and 111 online. 2022. Available at: https://digital.nhs.uk/data-and-information/publications/statistical/mi-potential-covid-19-symptoms-reported-through-nhs-pathways-and-111-online/latest

Nuffield Trust. NHS 111. 2022. Available at: www.nuffieldtrust.org.uk/resource/nhs-111#background

Robilotti E, Deresinski S, Pinsky BA. Norovirus. *Clinical microbiology reviews.* 2015;**28**(1):134-64.

Rodman J, Frost F, Jabukowski W. Using nurse hotline calls for disease surveillance. *Emerging infectious diseases.* 1998;**4**.

Rolland E, Moore KM, Robinson VA, McGuinness D. Using Ontario's "Telehealth" health telephone helpline as an early-warning system: a study protocol. *BMC health services research.* 2006;**6**:10-10.1186/1472-6963-6-10.

U.K. Health Security Agency. Remote Health Advice. 2022. Available at: https://www.gov.uk/government/publications/remote-health-advice-weekly-bulletins-for-2022

INTERNET SEARCH
DATA

Have fun and keep googling!

Larry Page, July 8th, 1988.

Can people's internet search habits tell us about the diseases they have and healthcare issues they face? It is natural that when we feel ill or have a medical complaint that we try to find out what is wrong with us and how to treat it. The internet is now the go-to place for quick and easy information. It is at our fingertips, with information being only a click away.

Imagine you invited friends round last night and had a jolly good time! The wine and conversation flowed. A bit too much actually. So this morning you wake up with a nasty headache! What is the best cure? You are not going to bother the doctor with this self inflicted minor health issue. How embarrassing to admit you can't handle your drink! Google it! Your search creates a digital record.

The power of large numbers
That individual query about your hangover is not much use to any researcher when it is performed in isolation. But there are a lot of people of earth; several billion. Many use the internet daily, often making multiple searches. I've made several just this morning. And although that hangover headache feels like the worst you have ever experienced, chances are that there are a large number of others who overdid it last night too, and are searching about how to deal with it this morning as well.

The sheer number of people there are, and the volume of searching being performed every day, means that patterns and trends soon begin to emerge and become apparent if you look for them. If you are suffering from some ailment the chances are that a corresponding number of people will be searching about it too.

Google Trends

The best known and most commonly used platform for research on internet search data is Google Trends. This chapter will concentrate on this resource, as it is the most popular for research purposes. This resource is based on a simple but nervelessness powerful idea. Basically, it shows what people are searching for on the internet and when. Google Trends was released in 2012, evolving from an earlier version called 'Google Insights for Search' which was released in 2008.

Interest in a particular search term is provided as a time series. Results are provided for specific search terms which can be single words or combinations of such words. A sample of web searches is used to generate this. Google Trends provides results in the form of a normalised index, with the period of most popular searching being given the value '100' against which searching at all other periods is calibrated against (Rogers, 2016). Not only does Google Trends provide pretty much real time up-to-date data, but it also provides a glimpse into searching in the past, with data being available from 2004 onwards.

Google Trends for 'hangover'

So let's return to our 'headache' after overindulging with the wine last night. When do other people search about hangovers and are there any patterns to see? On the following page is a graph using data from Google Trends showing the search results for 'hangover' for the U.K. for a 90 day period. The emphasis in this book is on disease outbreak detection and disease surveillance. Having a hangover is more a lifestyle condition than a disease. However, arguably alcohol abuse and addiction is a disease, and a pernicious one at that for those affected by it. Nevertheless, our hangover example shows the potential of Google Trends. Can you spot any patterns in 90 day searching? Surprise, surprise, there are weekly peaks in searching in the U.K., corresponding to the weekends. If you look at when people search in the 24 hour period it is in the morning. It is easy to conjecture that searching peaks when people wake up with that thick head.

Can we spot any long term trends apart from the weekend indulgence at the end of the working week? I would guess that peaks in alcohol consumption might correspond to football tournaments. Looking at data from 2004 this does not appear to be the case though. But clear peaks at Christmas and New Year periods are apparent. Again, this is probably not a surprise.

This simple example illustrates the usefulness of Google Trends in showing what people are searching for and when. Looking at such patterns is fun! Many hours can be spent looking for patterns and speculating on what causes them. The challenge lies in actually showing what the underlying cause for such patterns is. It is easy to speculate on possible reasons, but harder to actually demonstrate cause and effect.

It is easy to misinterpret patterns that appear. In our 'hangover' example there was a notable drop in searching during early 2020; just when the COVID-19 viral infection spread globally. During this period in the U.K. entertainment venues were closed and people often worked from home. So COVID-19 was a good thing! There was obviously a drop in excess alcohol misuse during this time! It appears that when people could not go out for a weekend binge they thus had fewer headaches and hangovers. However, it is generally agreed that alcohol consumption increased during this period and this has resulted in well reported alcohol related health problems (Killgore et al. 2021).

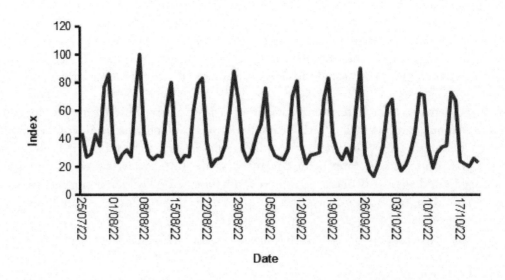

Above: Google Trends data on 'hangover' as a topic over 90 days for the U.K. July to October 2022. Note the weekly peaks. These peaks, beginning on the 29th of July occur every seven days. These are Sundays.

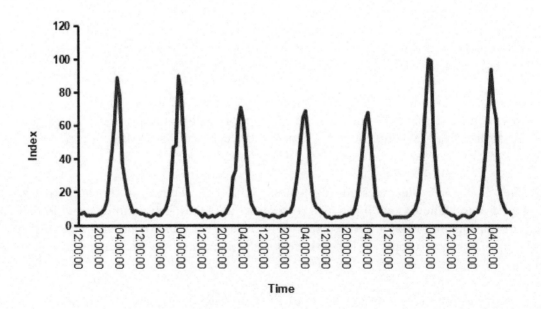

Above: Google Trends data on 'insomnia' as a topic for 7 days from the 18th of October 2022. Note that peak searching occurs in the early hours of the morning, approximately 4:00am.

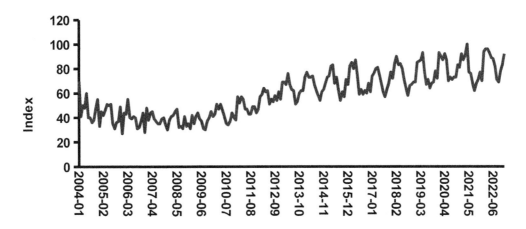

Above: Winter peaks are apparent in the monthly search volume for 'atopic dermatitis' (condition) for the U.K. Data from 2004 from Google Trends.

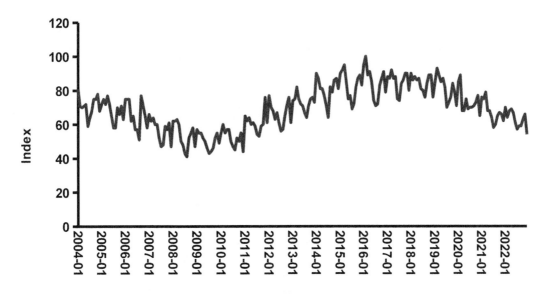

There are clear seasonal differences in the search volume for 'depression' (search term), with searching peaking in the Winter months and falling in the Summer. Note, the 'jagged' pattern to the Winter peak, with a notable decline in searching in December. Data for the U.K. From 2004 onwards.

Connecting internet searching with disease

Initially, the potential of Google Trends was quickly grasped by business people, who realised it could be used to study economic topics and maybe forecast trends in financial markets, and thus help make big money (Choi and Varian, 2012; Scharkow and Vogelsang, 2013; Preis et al. 2013). Epidemiologists, although less financially motivated, quickly realized the potential too. Does the level of internet searching on a specific healthcare condition or disease reflect the actual occurrence of that condition?

Maybe the earliest study looking at this was by Johnson et al. (2004). The authors obtained data from the 'healthlink' website on the number of access attempts made for influenza related articles. Then looking at Center for Disease Control data they looked at the relationship between the two. They found a moderately strong correlation suggesting that internet searching could be used to track influenza.

Another similar early study from Finland (Jormanainen et al. 2001) examined whether the frequency that medical doctors consulted guidelines on an online database was related to the reported cases of four diseases, including Lyme disease and pogosta disease.

Similarly, Hulth et al. (2009) examined internet searching about influenza on a Swedish medical website; Vårdguiden. Results for internet searching were compared with data on laboratory confirmed cases and with sentinel data from doctor surgeries for patients presenting with influenza like symptoms. The researchers used data on a variety of search terms including fever, headache, myalgia, cough, sore throat, coryza, and shortness of breath; all recognized signs of potential influenza. The researchers found that the intensity of searching for some of the influenza related terms closely matched the case data. They then went on to use the best search terms to develop a model which they could use to forecast future cases.

Pelat et al. (2009) examined searching with keywords related to three infectious conditions, influenza-like-illness, gastroenteritis, and chickenpox, then compared with clinical data from a sentinel medical network. They found certain keywords correlated extremely well.

Patterns in time

Particularly useful is that Google Trends makes periodic and seasonal trends more readily apparent. Sometimes such patterns were only previously suspected. Lyme disease was one of the first conditions where this was examined using Google Trends. It has long been known that reported cases mirrored the abundance of ticks in the environment. But Siefter et al. (2010) showed a strong seasonal pattern in searching on 'Lyme disease' and 'tick bite' which corresponded well to the seasonal pattern in reported cases, which mostly occur in Spring and Summer. Seasonal patterns in searching correspond to case numbers for other vector-borne conditions such as tick-borne encephalitis as well (Walker, 2018).

Conditions such as tick-borne diseases which are obviously seasonal in nature are an easy hit for researchers looking for similar seasonal patterns in internet searching. But some of the conditions where seasonal trends have become apparent were not so obvious. For example, examination of searching on 'knee pain' and 'knee swelling' showed greater search interest in Spring months. This is just when people were becoming more physically active after sedentary Winter months, and presumably went on to overdo things without sufficient training (Dewas and Sur, 2018). Infections of the urinary tract plague the lives of many women. However, no reliable data on the occurrence of this problem exists as no surveillance occurs. Is this condition more common at some periods of the year over others? Do urinary tract infections exhibit seasonality? This is the question French researchers set out to establish (Rossignol et al. 2013). They used Google Trends data on 'cystitis' and 'urinary tract infection' for France, Germany, Italy, the U.S., China, Australia and Brazil. They found that searching peaked in Summer months for France, Germany, the U.S., Italy and China, but in the austral Summer for Australia and Brazil. This is exactly as one would expect. Using a mathematical technique known as Fast Fourier Transformation, which basically examines which cyclical pattern fits the data best, they determined that searching cycled at one year frequencies.

Another example is provided by Yang et al. (2010), who were able to show variations in searching on the search term 'depression', demonstrating seasonal trends in searching by those in higher latitudes.

This ability of Google Trends to find previously hidden patterns demonstrates one of the key advantages of digital epidemiology; new sources of data, and new ways of examining data mean that our knowledge of healthcare conditions can be radically altered and improved.

Google Flu Trends

Being able to predict if and when a surge in influenza will occur is an important prize for epidemiologists to aim for. Can internet search data anticipate the annual upcoming surge in influenza? Polygren et al. (2008) used linear modelling along with internet search data and found they could predict increases in lab cases of influenza three weeks in advance of them occurring, and predict increases in mortality due to influenza five weeks in advance.

This research was built upon in Google Flu Trends, which can be considered as a form of Google Trends aiming specifically to forecast influenza. It was developed by the chief health strategist at Google, Roni Zeiger, and ran from 2008 to 2015. Using data on 50 million weekly search queries in the U.S., it assessed how well each fitted with official influenza-like-illness measures. The best ranking 45 search terms were then used in linear modelling to provide a forecast of likely future influenza levels. The research by Ginsberg et al. (2009) showed that using Google Trends data in this way for the U.S. allowed patterns in influenza to be estimated up to two weeks earlier than seen in official data from the Center for Disease Control. Just as important as the research, was that this research raised awareness of Google data and how it could be used to study epidemiology.

Initially the evidence seemed to show that Google Flu Trends (GFT) was pretty good at forecasting influenza. It was able to anticipate peaks during the epidemic that occurred in 2009 (Cook et al. 2011). Studies found that using Google Flu Trends improved short term forecasts for influenza. For example, Dugas (2013) utilized a type of model known as a generalized linear autoregressive moving average (GARMA), along with data from Google Flu Trends and found they could improve week ahead forecasts for influenza cases. Use of GFT proved better than other variables such as temperature or calendar week as added variables.

However, problems emerged when it became apparent that GFT overestimated the potential number of cases following the 2012 influenza season. Most notable was the study by Lazer et al. (2014), but also that of Pollett et al. (2016). Problems seem to have been caused by the symptom search terms used. A number of these were associated with conditions other than influenza. Surges in searching on these symptoms because of increases in other illnesses provided an overestimation of levels of influenza. Another problem was the effect of media coverage; search volumes were influenced by news coverage rather than increases in symptoms of illness. Google turned off Google Flu Trends in 2015, many argue prematurely. Later studies suggested that Google data could be effective in influenza forecasting (Osthus et al. 2019). Despite being turned off, data is however still obtainable from GFT (Google Flu Trends, 2022). However, debate over its utility continues.

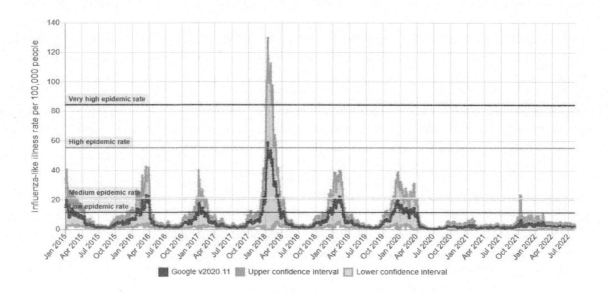

This shows data from the 'Flu Detector' system designed by University College London. It uses data from Google searches to provide an estimate of likely influenza-like-illness for England. This data is used by Public Health England to provide a forewarning of potential influenza outbreaks. Accessible from www.fludetector.cs.ucl.ac.uk

Google Dengue Trends

Dengue fever is one of those conditions which affects a staggeringly large number of people each year, but which because they live in the developing world remains relatively unheard of and ignored in the developed west. An estimated 400 million people become infected with dengue each year. Annually an estimated 25,000 die because of the condition (Roy and Bhattacharjee, 2021). Dengue fever is a viral infection, transmitted by female mosquitoes. Following infection symptoms begin to develop between 3 and 15 days (WHO, 2022). For most of those infected these symptoms are merely unpleasant and not serious. These include a fever, headaches, and a characteristic skin rash which can be most extensive. These symptoms begin to pass after about a week or so. But in a significant minority they instead worsen. Internal bleeding can then develop, leading to shock and eventual death.

A number of factors make dengue fever an ideal condition to test the effectiveness of surveillance using internet search data. Firstly, in many of the countries in which dengue occurs 'traditional' surveillance, that relying on the accurate reporting of cases by healthcare professionals, may be absent or limited. This could be due to geographical and communication problems. Remoteness and inhospitable terrain can hinder effective communication. However some of the countries affected are politically unstable. Many of them lack the financial resources to mount expensive epidemiological surveillance campaigns.

Another reason internet surveillance may be appropriate is that the incidence of dengue fever varies. Epidemics sometimes occur. Such variations do not occur in all the countries across its range, only in some. This variability makes predicting and forecasting the potential number of cases difficult. But it also makes any improvement in such prediction especially beneficial, as it can mean that additional resources can be designated to management in years of greatest need, and that preventative measures can be implemented with increased vigour.

In 2004 Google Dengue Trends (GDT) was developed by Google. Similarly to GFT, it used a range of search terms indicative of dengue fever, and then used these to forecast future cases. A study by Strauss et al. (2018) found that GDT was highly effective and data correlated well with official case numbers for Venezuela. Ho (2018) showed a relationship between Google Trends and dengue incidence in Manilla of the Philippines. A study by Husnayain (2019) in Indonesia found a high correlation between average case numbers of dengue fever and Google Trends data.

Advantages and disadvantages

The problems discussed with Google Flu Trends indicate one of the main problems with using internet search data to assess disease incidence in general. Are the patterns seen in internet searching actually reflective of incidence of the condition being studied on the ground? Internet searching can be influenced by a myriad of other factors. In the example of GFT, searches by those with other conditions but with symptoms shared with influenza made the GFT overestimate future case numbers. Many factors can influence the search patterns seen on Google Trends; celebrity gossip, news events unrelated to case numbers, or even music bands with song lyrics related to disease, can affect search patterns.

Another problem with using Google Trends data for disease surveillance, in particular if using search results for the name of a specific condition rather than symptoms, is that this presumes that the searcher knows what illness is affecting them. In some cases this might be fairly obvious, such as our example of 'hangover', but in other instances not so. Some conditions are difficult to diagnose. Use of internet search data appears to work best for those conditions where diagnosis is easy; with clear symptoms that are obvious even to those not medically trained. It appears less effective for conditions where diagnosis is problematic or where potential indicative symptoms are illusive. In some respects therefore, Google Trends results are dependent on the knowledge base of the population using it. This could vary between countries. This might not be related only to general level of education, but also the effectiveness of health promotion in a specific country.

A problem to date has been determining a structured methodology for such studies which allows results to be replicated. Results from Google Trends alter over time depending on recent and current search trends. A major peak in searching occurring today, will affect the results for corresponding searching for the past week, month, and year. Searching using Google 'search terms' or 'topic' categories results in slightly different results. Mavragani and Ochoa (2019) provide a framework for the standardization of studies using Google Trends and other search engines which should be consulted by anyone performing such research.

Despite these and other disadvantages it is easy to see why epidemiologists were quick to see the potential of internet search data. There are a number of potential advantages. For some conditions, internet search data could actually better reflect real on the ground levels of a disease or condition better than official reported case number data. Many conditions go unreported. People don't tend to go to the doctor with mild illnesses like common colds, instead treating themselves. In such cases data from internet searching might provide a good reflection of the numbers affected by such symptoms in a population, information not obtainable from official medical attendance records. Another example is provided by conditions which are potentially embarrassing condition, such as sexually transmitted conditions. Although methods exist to record and track what individual people search for on the internet, generally speaking, in most cases such searching is effectively anonymous.

A major advantage of using internet search data is that it is available instantaneously. Results are available in real-time (Carneiro and Mylonakis, 2009). There is no delay before records are available. This is particular important for conditions such as influenza where the situation can rapidly change and the most up-to-date picture of what is happening on the ground is required.

Internet search data, such as that from Google Trends, was used extensively throughout the initial stages of the COVID-19 pandemic. Studies showed a good correlation between levels of internet searching and the initial peak in cases, such as in the U.K. (Walker and Sulyok, 2020) Predictive models for COVID-19 were enhanced by the use of such data (Sulyok et al. 2020). Google provided datasets listing search trends on key COVID-19 symptoms (Google, 2022). Later studies including showing that Google searching was related to vaccination rates (Maugeri et al. 2022).

Another advantage is that internet search data can show the level of internet searching at a specific point in time. A literal interpretation of official data would make one think that all cases occur at 9am each day, or whatever hour they were released to the public. Sometimes official records are released only on a daily or weekly basis. As shown above with the examples such as 'insomnia', internet search data can show the specific hour of the day when searching is occurring. A final advantage is that internet search data is free with no cost, and easily accessible by all. You just need a computer with internet access.

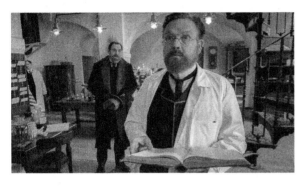

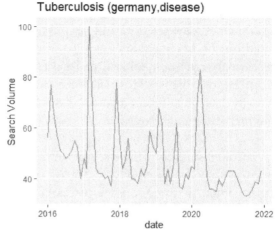

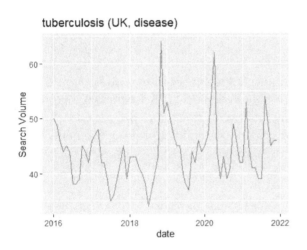

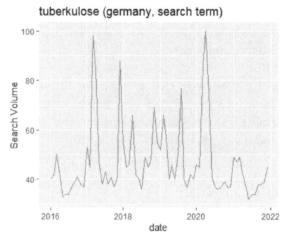

An effect of television on Google Trends? In March 2017 the main German broadcaster, the ARD, broadcast a fictional account of the work of the German scientists Rudolf Virchow, Emil Behring, Paul Ehrlich and Robert Koch, detailing their discoveries about tuberculosis. The program was a hit! Each episode attracted several million viewers. Study on Google Trends shows a clear peak in searching on 'tuberculosis' (disease)(name automatically generated by Google) and 'tuberkulose' (search term)(the German name) corresponding with the initial broadcast date in March 2017. For comparison, no such peak s in 2017 and 2018 occurred in a comparable search for the U.K. A program based on epidemiology is unlikely to be a hit in English speaking countries, where prime time television is mainly comprised of talent singing contests rather than documenting scientific progress. Note that there were peaks in Spring 2020 in both countries corresponding to the COVID-19 outbreak.

Where next?

Use of internet search data for research purposes is now common. Recent reviews cite large numbers of studies which have demonstrated that search data is related to disease incidence (Nuti et al. 2014). Such studies are easy and simple to perform if data on reported cases can be accessed. As pointed out by Mavragnani et al. (2018) in an excellent review, although studies relating searching to disease are common, what is missing is taking the next logical step and using such data to forecast and model disease. How can such methods be integrated with more traditional data sources? Can such data be combined with other variables such as meteorological data to meaningfully improve predictions of disease?

Also needing study is which search terms provide a best reflection of levels of each condition. Maybe the majority of studies so far use only a single obvious search term. Better results are likely to be obtained by using a range of search terms instead. The combination of such terms that together best reflect levels need to be found for each specific condition. Structured analysis to determine which search terms are most productive, and whether this changes over time will help future modelling work. Another avenue to explore is search terms related to weather or other external factors can improve disease forecasts. This has been investigated for some conditions such as Lyme disease (Kontowicz et al. 2022). Once this is done such data could be integrating into surveillance models.

An early warning system similar to Promed, which indicated when searching suddenly peaks and in which locations would be a logical next step for Google Trends data. A worldwide map showing localities where searching on the suite of symptoms indicative of dengue, plague, COVID-19, for example, with automatic notification of local authorities is a possibility to future advances.

REFERENCES

Carneiro HA, Mylonakis E. Google trends: a web-based tool for real-time surveillance of disease outbreaks. *Clinical infectious diseases.* 2009;**49**(10):1557-64.

Choi H, Varian H. Predicting the present with Google Trends. *Economic record.* 2012;**88**:2-9.

Cook S, Conrad C, Fowlkes AL, Mohebbi MH. Assessing Google flu trends performance in the United States during the 2009 influenza virus A (H1N1) pandemic. *Plos one.* 2011;**6**(8):e23610.

Dewan V, Sur H. Using google trends to assess for seasonal variation in knee injuries. *Journal of arthroscopy and joint surgery.* 2018;**5**(3):175-8.

Dugas AF, Jalalpour M, Gel Y, Levin S, Torcaso F, Igusa T, Rothman RE. Influenza forecasting with Google Flu Trends. *Plos one.* 2013;**8**(2):e56176.

Ginsberg J, Mohebbi MH, Patel RS, Brammer L, Smolinski MS, Brilliant L. Detecting influenza epidemics using search engine query data. *Nature.* 2009;**457**(7232):1012-4.

Google Flu Trends. Data. 2022. Available at: www.google.com/publicdata/explore?ds=z3bsqef7ki44ac_#!strail=false&bcs=d&nselm=h&rdim=country&ifdim=country&hl=en_US&dl=en_US&ind=false

Google LLC. Google COVID-19 Search Trends symptoms dataset. 2022. Available at: http://goo.gle/covid19symptomdataset.

Ho HT, Carvajal TM, Bautista JR, Capistrano JDR, Viacrusis KM, Hernandez LFT, Watanabe K. Using Google Trends to examine the spatio-temporal incidence and behavioral patterns of dengue disease: A case study in metropolitan Manila, Philippines. *Tropical medicine and infectious disease*. 2018;**3**(4):118.

Hulth A, Rydevik G, Linde A. Web queries as a source for syndromic surveillance. *Plos one*. 2009;**4**:e4378.

Husnayain A, Fuad A, Lazuardi L. Correlation between Google Trends on dengue fever and national surveillance report in Indonesia. *Global health action*. 2019;**12**(1):1552652.

Johnson HA, Wagner MM, Hogan WR, Chapman W, Olszewski RT, Dowling J, Barnas G. Analysis of web access logs for surveillance of influenza. *Medinfo*. 2004;**11**:1202-1206.

Jormanainen V, Jousimaa J, Kunnamo I, Ruutu P. Physicians' database searches as a tool for early detection of epidemics. *Emerging infectious diseases*. 2001;**7**(3):474.

Killgore WD, Cloonan SA, Taylor EC, Lucas DA, Dailey NS. Alcohol dependence during COVID-19 lockdowns. *Psychiatry research*. 2021;**296**:113676.

Kontowicz E, Brown G, Torner J, Carrel M, Baker KK, Petersen CA. Inclusion of environmentally themed search terms improves Elastic net regression nowcasts of regional Lyme disease rates. *Plos one*. 2022;**17**(3):e0251165.

Lazer D, Kennedy R, King G, Vespignani A. The parable of Google Flu: traps in big data analysis. *Science*. 2014;**343**(6176):1203-5.

Mavragani A, Ochoa G, Tsagarakis KP. Assessing the methods, tools, and statistical approaches in Google Trends research: systematic review. *Journal of medical internet research*. 2018;**20**(11):e9366.

Mavragani A, Ochoa G. Google Trends in infodemiology and infoveillance: methodology framework. *JMIR public health and surveillance*. 2019;**5**(2):e13439.

Maugeri A, Barchitta M, Agodi A. Using Google Trends to Predict COVID-19 Vaccinations and Monitor Search Behaviours about Vaccines: A Retrospective Analysis of Italian Data. *Vaccines*. 2022;**10**(1):119.

Nuti SV, Wayda B, Ranasinghe I, Wang S, Dreyer RP, Chen SI, Murugiah K. The use of google trends in health care research: a systematic review. *Plos one*. 2014;**9**(10):e109583.

Osthus D, Daughton AR, Priedhorsky RJP. Even a good influenza forecasting model can benefit from internet-based nowcasts, but those benefits are limited. *Plos computational*. 2019;**15**(2):e1006599.

Pelat C, Turbelin C, Bar-Hen A, Flahault A, Valleron AJ. More diseases tracked by using Google Trends. *Emerging infectious diseases*. 2009;**15**(8):1327.

Polgreen PM, Chen Y, Pennock DM, Nelson FD. Using internet searches for influenza surveillance. *Clinical infectious disease*. 2008;**47**:1443-1448.

Pollett S, Boscardin WJ, Azziz-Baumgartner E, Tinoco YO, Soto G, Romero C, et al. Evaluating Google Flu Trends in Latin America: important lessons for the next phase of digital disease detection. *Clinical infectious diseases*. 2017;64(1):34-41.

Preis T, Moat HS, Stanley HE. Quantifying trading behavior in financial markets using Google Trends. *Scientific reports*. 2013;**3**:1684.

Rogers S. What is Google Trends data and what does it mean. 2016. Google News Lab.

Rossignol L, Pelat C, Lambert B, Flahault A, Chartier-Kastler E, Hanslik T. A method to assess seasonality of urinary tract infections based on medication sales and google trends. *Plos one* 2013;**8**(10):e76020.

Roy SK, Bhattacharjee S. Dengue virus: epidemiology, biology, and disease aetiology. *Canadian journal of microbiology.* 2021;**67**(10):687-702.

Scharkow M, Vogelgesang J. Measuring the public agenda using search engine queries. *International journal of public opinion research* 2011;**23**(1):104-113.

Seifter A, Schwarzwalder A, Geis K, Aucott J. The utility of "Google Trends" for epidemiological research: Lyme disease as an example. *Geospatial health.* 2010;**4**(2):135-7.

Strauss RA, Castro JS, Reintjes R, Torres JR. Google dengue trends: An indicator of epidemic behavior. The Venezuelan Case. *International journal of medical informatics.* 2017;**104**:26-30.

Sulyok M, Ferenci T, Walker M. Google Trends Data and COVID-19 in Europe: Correlations and model enhancement are European wide. *Transboundary and emerging diseases.* 2021;**68**(4):2610-5.

Walker MD, Sulyok M. Online behavioural patterns for Coronavirus disease 2019 (COVID-19) in the United Kingdom. *Epidemiology and infection.* 2020;**148**.

Walker MD. Can Google be used to study parasitic disease? Internet searching on tick-borne encephalitis in Germany. *Journal of vector borne diseases.* 2018;**55**(4):327.

World Health Organisation (WHO). Dengue and Severe Dengue: Factsheet. 2022. Available at: www.who.int/news-room/fact-sheets/detail/dengue-and-severe-dengue

Yang AC, Huang NE, Peng CK, Tsai SJ. Do seasons have an influence on the incidence of depression? The use of an internet search engine query data as a proxy of human affect. *Plos one.* 2010;**5**(10):e13728.

NEWS MEDIA

News is something somebody doesn't want printed; all else is advertising.

William Randolph Hearst,
U.S. Newspaper magnate.

Open any newspaper and the chances are that somewhere within it there will be a medical or health related story. Such stories are staple topics of news media reporting, reflecting an inherent interest in such matters by the general public. News coverage on health and disease might cover the illnesses and ailments of famous people, discuss research developments, highlight problems such as long hospital waiting times, or describe individuals with unusual problems and who are seeking charitable funding for treatment. Editors want to sell copy; so they publish stories they think will interest us.

Crucially for the epidemiologist interested in disease surveillance, news reports might provide an indication about where a disease outbreak is occurring and how severe it is. The news media might report on an outbreak of an infectious condition occurring in a school, when there is a spike in case numbers of a disease locally, or might report on a notable individual such as a politician or celebrity who has succumbed to an infection. Such reports could provide a useful indicator of where a problem is arising and its extent.

Many news media sources
There are a large quantity of news sources. The print media, such as newspapers, are considered a traditional source of news. There are still over 1,200 daily newspapers in the U.S. alone, despite declines in recent years. There are 12 national daily newspapers in the U.K. and dozens of local daily newspapers. Added to this there are radio and television networks which provide news at regular intervals; the number of news broadcasts from these must run into the hundreds if not thousands each day.

The news media landscape has altered radically in the last 20 years because of the internet. Online news sources are now a major source of news for people (Olmstead et al. 2022). New news services and providers have appeared including Yahoo News and Google News. However, the websites of the traditional print media still dominate. For example, in the U.S. the websites of the New York Times and Washington Post remain amongst the most visited. Often email providers supply news stories as part of their email access. For example, stories from Yahoo News appear every time you access your emails. Google News is what is known as a 'news aggregator'; its online news services collect and collate news from around the world.

Can news media be used as a disease sentinel?

Resourceful epidemiologists have long realised that reports of disease in the news media could potentially provide a useful first indication of the geographical location of emerging health threats and disease outbreaks. A number of systems have utilised news media reports to provide an early warning of disease outbreaks; notable amongst them including 'HealthMap', the 'ProMED' newsletter , and the 'Global Public Health Intelligence Network'. These provide forewarning of the geographical location of potential disease outbreaks and highlight potential disease related problems.

Event based surveillance

The use of news reports as a indicator of such disease outbreaks is known as 'event based surveillance'. This term is used in the literature to denote the use of informal sources of information, such as online news reports, email, social media 'gossip', or other non-standard recording sources to identify and quantify potential disease problems (WHO, 2014). The advantage of using such data, is that although it may be unreliable and of uncertain veracity, it provides a quicker indication of potential outbreaks and their extent than the standard and official methods of disease surveillance.

Is there a relationship between the amount of news coverage and disease incidence?

However, relatively few studies have tried to quantitatively assess the relationship between media coverage and disease incidence. Any link probably depends on the nature of the disease involved, and is likely to be strongest for rare and severe conditions which have the 'fear' factor, such as Ebola virus.

One study which examined whether there was such a link looked at newspaper coverage in response to a press release about mumps released by the U.K. Health Protection Agency (Olowokure, 2007). The study examined the effect this had on the notification of cases of mumps within the 15 to 24 year age group in the west midlands of England and Wales. Notification of mumps increased after publication of the press release, and the related subsequent increase in newspaper coverage this caused. However the number of media reports the press release generated was low; the maximum being 13 in any of the time periods examined in the study, meaning that drawing any firm conclusions was difficult.

Another study examined the relationship between media coverage and reporting of gastroenteritis during a cryptosporidiosis outbreak in north west England (Elliot et al. 2016). This found a relationship between the distribution of a 'boil water notice' by a local water company and presentation of suspected cases to local medical practises.

Zhang et al. (2020) used the LexisNexis database which lists media reports to assess how well media coverage covered Zika virus and dengue fever outbreaks, both vector borne conditions common in India and Brazil. A selected number of national media sources and two local newspapers were monitored using the LexisNexis resource for each country. Articles were assessed and categorised using text mining techniques. Local newspapers proved to be best correlated with dengue fever cases in India, while in Brazil national media was better for Zika with the number of media reports mirroring official case numbers. The results maybe emphasise that different methods are potentially best for different specific conditions. However, another study failed to find any relation between news coverage and dengue fever in India (Villanes et al. 2018)

Using news reports to predict whether a disease outbreak will occur

Can information gathered from news media sources be used to forecast where disease outbreaks will occur and when case numbers might peak? Kim and Ahn (2021) examined news media coverage on a multitude of diseases across the globe and examined whether this could be used to predict future occurrence. The number of reports on each condition in each country were obtained from the media platform MedIsys. Different machine learning models were used to examine the data, with the effectiveness of each one being contrasted. The authors examined 115,279 articles. However, no comparison with how well forecasts mirrored actual reported case numbers was made.

In an earlier study by the same authors (Kim and Ahm, 2019), whether the number of news reports on influenza could be used to forecast likely future rates using the machine learning method support vector machines was examined. The study compared forecasted results with data from the Center for Disease Control on influenza as the official source for comparison.

Li et al. (2021) used the Sina Network Opinion Surveillance System (SNOSS), a platform which monitors online news sources, and with modelling found that data from this resource could be used to anticipate influenza levels in China.

SYSTEMS FOR MEDIA MONITORING

ProMED mail

This email alerts service collates reports of disease from a variety of sources, including online news reports. It acts as a news service for epidemiologists, informing them of potential outbreaks and so is worthy of mention in this section. This was one of the first news based disease alerts to be established, initially being released in 1994 by the International Society of Infectious Diseases. It continues to be widely used today. It is now well established and has proven successful at informing the epidemiological community about a range of serious outbreaks. Good examples where ProMed has been useful in raising awareness of novel diseases include its reporting on the Middle East Respiratory Syndrome Coronavirus (MERS-CoV), first identified in 2012 (Pollack et al. 2017), and Crimean-Congo haemorrhagic fever (Ince et al. 2014).

EpiSpider

EpiSpider is the computer application which works with ProMED mail to take location information from reports and then plot them on Google Maps. This helps visualize the geographical location of outbreaks in a more readily comprehensible format (Tolentino et al. 2007).

MedIsys

This is an early warning system for a range of health related issues including food borne and infectious disease. It automatically assesses media reports, providing summaries and analysis. A user can perform a search for a specific health problem, and filter results for specific geographical locations and languages. MedIsys is part of the European Unions Europe Media Monitor and is closely connected with the NewsDesk system. The range of media examined by this system is large; with over 3,600 sources including newspapers and governmental websites being used (Linge et al. 2011).

Websites are 'scraped' automatically for keywords indicative of disease, which are then used to produce the overall summaries. A range of infectious and vector borne conditions are included on the MedIsys system (Mantero et al. 2011). Real time surveillance can be performed with alerts being produced showing location, and the number of reported cases of a condition. Related is the News-Brief website, which is a more general media analysis portal which details the trending news stories of the day. A study examining how well MedIsys compared to official sources that record cases of food borne illness found that MedIsys compared favourably (Rortais et al. 2010).

Linge et al. (2011) describes patterns in media coverage relating to two outbreaks using data from the MedIsys system. The first was an outbreak of legionellosis in Spain in October 2010 which resulted in a spike in media reporting in Spain on related search terms. The second example is of an entero-haemorrhagic *Escherichia coli* outbreak in Germany, which affected several thousand people in May 2011. A peak in media coverage was correlated with official case number data.

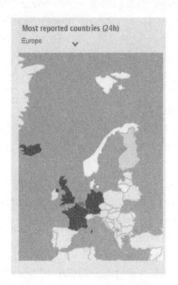 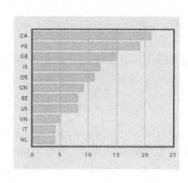 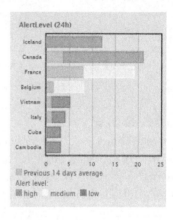

**Figures from the NewsBrief website, the sister site of MedIsys,
showing articles on avian influenza over a 24 hour period in July 2022.
This indicates potential alerts for Canada and Iceland.**

Global Public Health Intelligence Network
The Global Public Health Intelligence Network (GPHIN) monitors online news, categorising reports in order to identify likely disease outbreaks (Dion et al. 2015).

BioCaster
Another automatic news and media monitoring system is BioCaster (Collier et al. 2012). Originally running from 2006 to 2012, it was later re-launched as part of a collaboration between the University of Cambridge and McGill University in Canada. It is part of the EPI-AI project. The system uses natural language processing to detect news articles mentioning potentially disease related topics.

HealthMap

HealthMap is a more graphic map based system, which collates reports from a variety of sources including from the news media, to show in map form locations where disease outbreaks might be occurring (Freifeld et al. 2008). This website monitors news sites such as Google News, as well as more conventional sources, to provide the geographical location of potential disease outbreaks.

A study examining whether news reports from HealthMap were related to cases of cholera following the Haitian earthquake of January 2010 found that the volume of HealthMap reports was well correlated with official data and preceded them by up to two weeks (Chunara et al. 2012). Later, HealthMap proved its worth in 2014 when it successfully tracked the emergence of an Ebola epidemic that occurred in West Africa in that year. Now a special version of HealthMap is available especially conceived with Ebola in mind, which provides current and recent posts from news media organisations from the locations where Ebola could occur.

A study by Majumber et al. (2015) using HealthMap reports showed that media reports detailing control measures were associated with a subsequent decline in Ebola. Thus media reporting can be actively used during disease outbreaks to change behaviours and help control the situation, as well as providing the potential to identify disease hotspots as they are occurring.

EpiNews, a platform for processing informal and online news stories related to disease can use HealthMap reports (Ghosh et al. 2017). Using mathematical modelling to look at the temporal patterns in reporting, EpiNews can use information on the volume of news related stories to determine whether there is a potential outbreak occurring. Ghosh et al. (2017) gave examples for a range of seasonal condition including salmonellosis case counts in the U.S and hand foot and mouth disease in China.

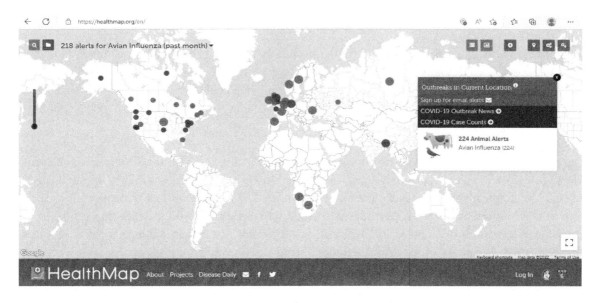

The HealthMap homepage, here showing avian influenza reports globally.

General News Media Systems

Epidemiologists are not the only ones interested in what the media is covering. There are many business reasons for monitoring the news, such as keeping an eye on the competition, spotting trends in the markets, or anticipating market demand. An innovative fashion retailer would do well to monitor the media for reports on outfits worn by celebrities, for example.

Thus there are a number of general media monitoring systems. Examples include:
- Lexis-Nexis (2019), formerly Nexis Uni (2018)
- Factiva (2022)
- Infotrac (2018)
- Newspaper.com (2018)

These have been little used for epidemiological purposes, but have the potential to be so. The study by Zhang et al. (2020) which used Lexis-Nexis, has already been described. In a non epidemiological study, Weaver and Bimber (2008) compared searching effectiveness of Google News and Lexis-Nexis, finding great variability in the search success between the two. Lexis-Nexis missed many stories reported elsewhere.

An example of media coverage and disease: H1N1 'swine flu' influenza

The best recent example where the relationship between media coverage and corresponding disease occurrence has been examined is provided by the H1N1 'swine flu' influenza pandemic of 2009. A content analysis of newspaper coverage in the U.K. found that media coverage followed a similarly bimodal pattern as reported cases (Hilton and Hunt, 2011) Although media reporting showed a similar pattern as disease cases, the periods of greatest media interest occurred in the Spring, whereas the number of confirmed cases actually peaked in Autumn. The authors believed this reflected the initially grave concerns about the virulence of this pathogen, which later proved unfounded.

Similarly in the U.K., the number of media enquiries about H1N1 made to Public Health Wales during the 2009 epidemic was found to correspond to the Spring and Autumn peaks in reported cases (Keramarou et al. 2011). Another study examined weekly news coverage about H1N1, and found a relationship between reporting of cases and media interest related to schools, albeit not a strong one (Olowokure, 2012).

Dutch media coverage was found to be most intensive in the initial and end stages of the epidemic (de Lange, 2013). A content analysis of the main Dutch newspapers and TV coverage on H1N1, was able to demonstrate that news coverage was linked to key events in the progression of the disease in the Netherlands. Media coverage increased when the first Dutch death was reported, for example (Vasterman and Ruigrok, 2013). Similar as to what was seen in the U.K., it was found that although most hospitalisations and deaths occurred in Autumn, the greatest amount of newspaper coverage on H1N1 occurred in late Spring.

The only other study to suggest that media interest preceded official recording of cases assessed media coverage on H1N1 in several European countries and found that media interest in H1N1 peaked well before corresponding peaks in case numbers (Reinjes et al 2016). An advantage of this study was the relatively large numbers of media articles able to be examined for each country, meaning a good reflection of true media interest was obtained.

Does news coverage precede disease?

The evidence that there is a relationship between disease incidence and social media usage and internet searching is good. Numerous studies have demonstrated that trends in social media usage and internet searching precede official reported case numbers of disease.

However, whether a similar relationship occurs between news media coverage and disease reporting is uncertain. It is unclear whether news media reporting precedes reported cases or whether they react to them. As shown by Linge et al. (2011), although the volume of media reporting was related to the number of enterohemorrhagic *Escherichia coli* cases seen in Germany during an outbreak, the media reporting occurred sometime after recording of cases officially.

The relationship between media reporting and disease incidence could well be location specific. For example, it could well be the case that in remote areas of the globe where official communication channels are poor, journalists may be able to report quicker than official channels can identify, test, and subsequently report disease through official channels. This could well be especially the case given today's technological progress, with posting online being able to be done pretty much instantaneously. However, it may be that in more developed countries, where possibly greater emphasis is placed on ensuring accurate reporting, journalists prefer to react to officially confirmed cases rather than preceding them.

Advantages and disadvantages

There are a number of potential advantages to using news media to study trends in disease incidence:

- **More sources:** There are probably more journalists looking for stories than there are epidemiologists searching for disease outbreaks. Although not scientifically trained, at least journalists tend to be educated professionals and trained investigators. Thus, the reports they write can be considered as somewhat reliable. Journalists have a vested interest in providing news that is correct and can be verified; their jobs are worth it. This means journalists can extend the traditional disease surveillance net made up solely by epidemiologists considerably.

- **Speed:** Traditional surveillance can be slow, being held up by delays in routine administration. A journalist values speed and wants to publish stories quickly, preferably before they are scooped by others. Stories can appear hours after being written on online portals and blogs, and even in print only a few days after being written. There is a trade off here though with reliability and accuracy.

However there are also a number of potential disadvantageous to this information source:

- **Other factors influence news coverage:** All because a news article contains mention of a disease, does not mean there is an outbreak of that condition. For example, a celebrity might reveal in an interview they fear they have some condition, hoping to generate public sympathy and interest, or to promote a book or new television series. Coverage about Lyme disease for example, is skewed by celebrities stating that they have the condition

(Walker, 2021). A disease might be mentioned in the news media for issues unrelated to its incidence, such as a new treatment having been developed against it.

- **Accuracy:** As mentioned above, with potentially untrained individuals providing reports comes the risk of reports not being entirely accurate. Journalists might report on suspected cases which subsequently turn out to be false or simply rumours. Medical professionals are not immune to mistakes. But at least if proper official procedures are followed, with a requirement for testing before confirmation, then the chances of recorded data being accuracy are far greater.

- **Epidemiology echo-chamber:** Often the sources journalists use for health related stories are epidemiologists themselves (De Semir et al. 1998), or government officials, or simply other journalists. If a surveillance organization releases a press release about a disease outbreak, that will be picked up by the media. It can thus be that the news media is simply amplifying officially released information that epidemiologists already know about.

- **Disease is not important:** Although it is difficult for disease scientists to comprehend, not everyone is fascinated by disease. Journalists and editors might be interested in disease as a potential story, but it is not there main priority or motivation in life. Even amongst local newspapers, a case of a suspected serious disease might not find room due to other 'more important' local stories concerning local politicians. On a national level a celebrity couple who split up might be considered more newsworthy than a new pandemic in some quarters of the press.

- **Disruption:** Where normal journalism is disrupted, in times of war for instance, then reports of disease are likely to be missed. Journalists are unlikely to be able to travel and report freely and thus disease outbreaks could be missed.

- **Waning interest:** There could conceivably be much news media interest when a disease outbreak is first identified. But over time media interest wanes. An example is provided by the level of media interest in the H1N1 'swine flu' influenza outbreak in the U.K., where initially high media interest quickly declined (Hilton and Hunt, 2011). More important is the next big story. There are doubts as to whether media coverage reflect the changing trends and patterns in disease occurrence over time. There is likely to be a large initial peak in reporting, followed by a steady decline in reports.

- **News coverage varies:** The amount of media varies geographically making comparison difficult. For example, a developed country like Germany has many media outlets and many newspapers. A poorer country like Chad, has far fewer. Thus knowledge of local situations is required and taken into consideration. Country comparison is hardly possible. Can disease outbreaks be studied at a level smaller than the national level? This is unknown and requires investigation.

- **Disease is often not an event:** News needs events. Although to the individual involved becoming infected with a disease is very much a life event, it is not necessary one of interest to journalists or the wider public. Often the number of cases of a disease can rise in a population almost surreptitiously, unnoticed, and in a un-newsworthy fashion. News requires sudden large impact events. Thus, only the most severe and life affecting of disease outbreaks are likely to be well covered, such as Ebola. The more 'quiet' diseases, such as influenza, which kill unnoticed and affect much larger numbers of people are reported comparatively less.

COVID-19 and the news

The COVID-19 pandemic dominated the news agenda worldwide in the Spring of 2020. In the U.K. the virus received blanket news coverage out of all relation to the initially small number of cases. Initial research of the American PEW surveys suggests there was a large increase in interest in news coverage amongst the general public during the crisis, especially through legacy media (Casero-Ripollés 2020).

This is reflected by sources from private media monitoring services, such as the COVID-19 dashboard established by the CISION media group. This shows the volume of media articles mentioning COVID-19. This was initially extremely large, which is understandable given the unprecedented nature of the pandemic. However, media interest declined in later months. As pointed out by Pearman et al. (2021) this decline in media coverage was despite the fact that the actual number of cases and the number of deaths was increasing.

Much of the research examining COVID-19 media coverage has concentrated on performing content analysis, rather than looking at whether such coverage is related to case numbers. A number of studies have suggested that trends in internet search interest on COVID-19 are related to media coverage rather than incidence. For example, Szmuda et al. (2021) suggested that internet searching was more closely related to WHO media alerts than case numbers. However, whether WHO media alerts reflect media coverage more generally was not examined. Liu et al. (2020) found that as media coverage increased, the number of cases declined in local areas of China. This suggests as reports increased, there was increased heeding of control measures.

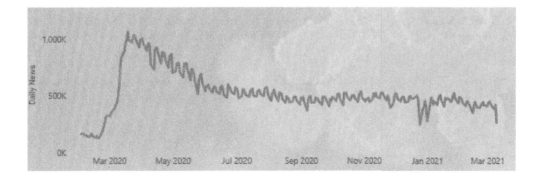

The private media monitoring company CISION produced a COVID-19 dashboard showing the number of media articles mentioning COVID-19 throughout the pandemic. It shows the initial peak in the Spring of 2020 followed by a gradual waning of interest.

99

What next?

Here, we have looked at whether news reporting can be used to identify when and where disease outbreaks are happening, and also whether there is any relationship between news media coverage and disease incidence. However, identification of outbreaks is only one potential use of the news media for those engaged in the health sciences. Neglected here is the great potential the media offers in terms of health education. Health communication is an important discipline in its own right (Briggs and Hallin, 2016). News media coverage helps inform the public about disease threats and can help improve health literacy. There is good evidence that health communication can change habits, leading to healthy lives (Wakefield et al. 2010). Little research has examined the effectiveness of media coverage on changing habits and behaviours in response to infectious disease outbreaks.

The question as to whether news media can be used to identify outbreaks is still uncertain. Ironically, as technology progresses further, the potential of news media as a potential data source for epidemiologists may disappear. Fast progress is being made on the development of semi-automatic, and increasingly even totally automatic, news writing programs which scan potential news sources and write copy without an actual physical reporter being required. News is beginning to transcend geographical boundaries making identifying locations of outbreaks increasingly difficult. Even systems monitoring disease outbreaks using news media rarely do so at the local level, most at the national.

REFERENCES

Briggs CL, Hallin DC. Making health public: how news coverage is remaking media, medicine, and contemporary life. London: Routledge, 2016.

Casero-Ripollés A. Impact of Covid-19 on the media system. Communicative and democratic consequences of news consumption during the outbreak. *El profesional de la información.* 2020;**29**(2):e290223.

Chunara R, Andrews JR, Brownstein JS. Social and news media enable estimation of epidemiological patterns early in the 2010 Haitian cholera outbreak. *American journal of tropical medicine and hygiene.* 2012;**86**(1):39-45.

Collier N, Doan S, Kawazoe A, Goodwin RM, Conway M, Tateno Y, Ngo QH, Dien D, Kawtrakul A, Takeuchi K, Shigematsu M. BioCaster: detecting public health rumors with a Web-based text mining system. *Bioinformatics.* 2008;**24**(24):2940-1.

de Lange M, Meijer A, Friesema IH, Donker GA, Koppeschaar CE, Hooiveld M, Ruigrok N, van der Hoek W. Comparison of five influenza surveillance systems during the 2009 pandemic and their association with media attention. *BMC public health.* 2013;**13**(1):1-0.

De Semir V, Ribas C, Revuelta G. Press releases of science journal articles and subsequent newspaper stories on the same topic. *Journal of the American medical association.* 1998;**280**(3):294-5.

Dion M, AbdelMalik P, Mawudeku A. Big data: big data and the global public health intelligence network (gphin). *Canada communicable disease report.* 2015;**41**(9):209.

Elliot AJ, Hughes HE, Astbury J, Nixon G, Brierley K, Vivancos R, Inns T, Decraene V, Platt K, Lake I, O'Brien SJ. The potential impact of media reporting in syndromic surveillance: an example using a possible Cryptosporidium exposure in North West England, August to September 2015. *Eurosurveillance.* 2016;**13**:21(41).

Factiva. 2018. Available at: https://www.dowjones.com/products/factiva/

Freifeld CC, Mandl KD, Reis BY, Brownstein JS. HealthMap: global infectious disease monitoring through automated classification and visualization of internet media reports. *Journal of the American medical informatics association.* 2008;**15**(2):150-7.

Ghosh S, Chakraborty P, Nsoesie EO, Cohn E, Mekaru SR, Brownstein JS, Ramakrishnan N. Temporal topic modeling to assess associations between news trends and infectious disease outbreaks. *Scientific reports.* 2017;**7**(1):1-2.

Hilton S, Hunt K. UK newspapers' representations of the 2009–10 outbreak of swine flu: one health scare not over-hyped by the media?. *Journal of epidemiology and community health.* 2011; **65**(10): 941-6.

Ince Y, Yasa C, Metin M, Sonmez M, Meram E, Benkli B, Ergonul O. Crimean-Congo hemorrhagic fever infections reported by ProMED. *International journal of infectious diseases.* 2014;**26**:44-6.

InfoTrac Newsstand. 2018. Available at: https://www.gale.com/c/infotrac-newsstand

Keramarou M, Cottrell S, Evans MR, Moore C, Stiff RE, Elliott C, Thomas DR, Lyons M, Salmon RL. Two waves of pandemic influenza A (H1N1) 2009 in Wales–the possible impact of media coverage on consultation rates, April–December 2009. *Eurosurveillance.* 2011;**16**(3):19772.

Kim J, Ahn I. Infectious disease outbreak prediction using media articles with machine learning models. *Scientific reports.* 2021;**11**(1):1-3.

Kim J, Ahn I. Weekly ILI patient ratio change prediction using news articles with support vector machine. *BMC bioinformatics.* 2019;**20**(1):1-6.

Lexis-Nexis. 2018. Available at: https://www.lexisnexis.com/communities/academic/w/wiki/30.lexisnexis-academic-general-information.aspx

Li J, Sia CL, Chen Z, Huang W. Enhancing influenza epidemics forecasting accuracy in China with both official and unofficial online news articles, 2019–2020. *International journal of environmental research and public health.* 2021;**18**(12):6591.

Linge JP, Verile M, Tanev H, Zavarella V, Fuart F, van der Goot E. Media monitoring of public health threats with medisys. *C. WILLIAM, CWR. WEB-STER, D. BALAHUR,* et al. 2012:17-31.

Liu N, Chen Z, Bao G. Role of media coverage in mitigating COVID-19 transmission: Evidence from China. *Technological forecasting and social change.* 2021;**163**:120435.

Majumder MS, Kluberg S, Santillana M, Mekaru S, Brownstein JS. 2014 Ebola outbreak: media events track changes in observed reproductive number. *Plos currents.* 2015;**7**.

Mantero J, Belyaeva J, Linge JP. How to maximise event-based surveillance web-systems the example of ECDC/JRC collaboration to improve the performance of MedISys. Luxembourg: Publications Office of the European Union. 2011.

Newspapers.com. 2018. Available at: https://go.newspapers.com/welcome?xid=767&gclid=Cj0KCQiAmafh-BRDUARIsACOKERO4PtO4FBuYZuILilnBvTeBoKtWS6I2txdBOkPPRFWjdAyB7rwonB4aAkbiEALw_wcB

Nexis Uni. 2019. Available at: https://www.lexisnexis.com/en-us/support/nexis-uni/default.page

Olmstead K, Mitchell A, Rosenstiel T. Navigating news online: Where people go, how they get there and what lures them away. Pew Research Center. 2020. Available at: https://www.pewresearch.org/wp-content/uploads/sites/8/legacy/NIELSEN-STUDY-Copy.pdf

Olowokure B, Odedere O, Elliot AJ, Awofisayo A, Smit E, Fleming A, Osman H. Volume of print media coverage and diagnostic testing for influenza A (H1N1) pdm09 virus during the early phase of the 2009 pandemic. *Journal of clinical virology.* 2012;**55**(1):75-8.

Olowokure B, Clark L, Elliot AJ, Harding D, Fleming A. Mumps and the media: changes in the reporting of mumps in response to newspaper coverage. *Journal of epidemiology and community health.* 2007;**61**(5):385-8.

Pearman O, Boykoff M, Osborne-Gowey J, Aoyagi M, Ballantyne AG, Chandler P, Daly M, Doi K, Fernández-Reyes R, Jiménez-Gómez I, Nacu-Schmidt A. COVID-19 media coverage decreasing despite deepening crisis. *Lancet planetary health.* 2021;**5**(1):e6-7.

Pollack MP, Pringle C, Madoff LC, Memish ZA. Latest outbreak news from ProMED-mail: novel coronavirus–Middle East. *International journal of infectious disease.* 2013;**17**(2):e143-4.

Reintjes R, Das E, Klemm C, Richardus JH, Keßler V, Ahmad A. "Pandemic Public Health Paradox": time series analysis of the 2009/10 Influenza A/H1N1 epidemiology, media attention, risk perception and public reactions in 5 European countries. *Plos one;* 2016:**11**(3).

Rortais A, Belyaeva J, Gemo M, Van der Goot E, Linge JP. MedISys: An early-warning system for the detection of (re-) emerging food-and feed-borne hazards. *Food research international.* 2010;**43**(5):1553-6.

Szmuda T, Ali S, Hetzger TV, Rosvall P, Słoniewski P. Are online searches for the novel coronavirus (COVID-19) related to media or epidemiology? A cross-sectional study. *International journal of infectious diseases.* 2020;**97**:386-90.

Tolentino MH. Scanning the emerging infectious diseases horizon - visualizing ProMED emails using EpiSPIDER. *Advances in disease surveillance.* 2007;**2**:169.

Vasterman PL, Ruigrok N. pandemic alarm in the Dutch media: Media coverage of the 2009 influenza A (H1N1) pandemic and the role of the expert sources. *European journal of communication.* 2013;**28**(4):436-53.

Villanes A, Griffiths E, Rappa M, Healey CG. Dengue fever surveillance in India using text mining in public media. *The American journal of tropical medicine and hygiene.* 2018;**98**(1):181.

Wakefield MA, Loken B, Hornik RC. Use of mass media campaigns to change health behaviour. *Lancet.* 2010; **376**(9748):1261-71.

Walker MD. The portrayal of Lyme Disease by a public service broadcaster. *Journal of communication in healthcare.* 2021;**14**(4):303-11.

Weaver DA, Bimber B. Finding news stories: a comparison of searches using LexisNexis and Google News. *Journalism and mass communication quarterly.* 2008;**85**(3):515-30.

World Health Organisation (WHO). *Early detection, assessment and response to acute public health events: Implementation of early warning and response with a focus on event-based surveillance,* 2014.

Zhang Y, Ibaraki M, Schwartz FW. Disease surveillance using online news: Dengue and Zika in tropical countries. *Journal of biomedical informatics.* 2020;**102**:103374.

ONLINE SURVEYING

Our survey said......

Family Fortunes (U.K.), Family Feud (U.S.A).

What better way to find something out than to ask? Surveying the public to ascertain their opinion has a long history, predating modern technological developments in computing. For example, the first attempt at a national census took place in the U.K. in March 1801, when overseers of the poor were tasked with recording the number of people living in each household. However, the 1841 census is generally agreed to be the first effective modern day census with more detailed records being collected.

The use of computers to aid such census and survey collection has a long history. A system of using machine counted punched cards was developed by the American Herman Hollerith and was used as early as 1890 in the U.S. census of that year. In fact, it could be argued that it was the need for public surveying that drove the invention of computers in the first place. One of the companies begun by Hollerith went on to become part of International Business Machines, IBM, in 1924.

As technology has progressed the methods and scope of such surveying has changed dramatically. Today, surveys can be developed and designed by anyone. A range of online services exist to promote this. The widespread use of email and the internet has made it increasingly easy to reach large numbers of people, without needing significant financial or time investment, as is required for postal or face to face surveying.

Using email: A questionnaire of ill mountain bike racers

Email offers a free and easy method to contact large numbers of people quickly. It was one of the first technologies of the internet age that provided epidemiologists with the ability to contact those affected by disease and ascertain basic information about disease outbreaks.

Use of email questionnaires initially proved useful when investigating small scale disease outbreaks, and meant that the contact details of those potentially affected could be easily obtained. One of the earliest examples where email was used for such disease outbreak investigation was at a leptospirosis outbreak at a university campus in Hawaii (Gaynor et al. 2007).

Another example is provided by a campylobacteriosis outbreak, which occurred in June 2007, following a mountain bike race in British Colombia, Canada (Chester et al. 2011). Mountain biking is an adventurous undertaking, not for the faint hearted. Typically races are run over rough terrain; often involving descents down steep banks, and traversing rocks and vegetation. Depending on the weather conditions there can be large amounts of mud!

Following the event in British Colombia a number of riders began to fall ill. The first reports of illness were reported only two days following the event. Laboratory investigations concluded that campylobacter was the cause; this was ascertained only nine days following the race.

Those tasked with investigating the outbreak decided to utilize a web forum for mountain bike riders in addition to creating their own bespoke questionnaire sent using email. Luckily as part of signing up for the event, participants had to provide their email addresses. This provided the epidemiologists investigating the outbreak with the ability to contact many of those who could have been involved in the race and many who had been affected by campylobacteriosis.

The web forum itself also proved a useful source of information, with over 50 posts discussing the mystery illness outbreak and what could have caused it. The online questionnaire was designed within 48 hours. The results provided useful information on participants, such as that most were male and of Canadian nationality. Of 549 race participants it was found that 225, thus 42%, had fallen ill. 53% of those asked to participate in surveying provided answers, which was considered a higher response rate than that obtained usually through more traditional forms of surveying. The most likely cause of the outbreak appears to have been inadvertent ingestion of contaminated mud!

Telephone surveying

Of course surveying can be conducted using the telephone. A study by Malone et al. (2008) examined the feasibility of conducting nationwide telephone surveys about influcnza and whether the results could enhance other forms of sentinel monitoring. Over 7,000 people were contacted over seven survey rounds. Promising results were obtained, providing a useful picture of the influenza situation nationally.

Technological progress since this time means that telephone surveying today offers more potential to obtain such data. The process of telephoning can now be automated, with telephone calls being sent and data collected without the need for actual telephonists, instead using pre-recorded messages.

Online surveying

As the internet developed a range of online companies providing survey templates allowing the quick and easy development of individual surveys came into existence. Such online surveying developed rapidly along with the growth of the internet (Evans and Mathur, 2018). Perhaps the most well known tool for developing online surveys is SurveyMonkey (2023), which was started in 1999 by Ryan and Chris Finley. However, many other companies exist, including Qualtrics which began in 2002.

Such online surveys soon began to be used to investigate disease outbreaks. For example, a 2007 outbreak of campylobacter in Stockholm, Sweden, was investigated using such an online survey (de Johg and Anker, 2008).

In an early example of the use of the web to undertake disease surveillance in a targetted manner, Surgiura et al. (2010) developed a questionnaire asking participants to a G8 economic conference at Izumo city, Japan, about symptoms of illness they were experiencing. Six symptoms were asked about, likely to indicate either a bioterrorist attack or an outbreak of an infectious disease. Surveying took part daily with participants being messaged and urged to take part. An initial survey was trialled over the web and telephone, and later refined and implemented at the G8 summit meeting itself.

Estimating H1N1 cases

During the Winter of 2009, the H1N1 influenza virus spread across England causing influenza-like-illness. How many people were affected? Brooks-Pollack et al. (2011) described the 'flusurvey', an online questionnaire that was promoted in the media. Participants were asked to sign up and provide health information and specifically whether they were experiencing any symptoms indicative of influenza. The survey ran from July 2009 to March 2010.

The data collected was used to estimate the number of people affected; producing an estimate of 1.1 million symptomatic cases. This was 40% greater than the previous estimate using data from consultations to medical practitioners. The internet survey was able to reach groups who did not access healthcare and thus were not recorded in sentinel medical practise data.

The Great Influenza Survey: De Grote Griepmeting

A good example of an online survey used to monitor disease is provided by 'De Grote Griepmeting', or to use the English name 'the Great Influenza Survey' (Vandendijck et al. 2013). This proved a forerunner for other European systems including 'Influenzanet'.

The Great Influenza Survey started in 2005, with participants being asked to complete online surveys detailing any symptoms they had. For example they were asked whether they were suffering from fever. The survey was limited to the Flemish part of Belgium initially, as it was in Dutch.

Running over several years, the number of participants varied annually from 3,135 to 11,579. Study of the data showed a strong correlation of those found with influenza-like-illness in the surveys with sentinel medical data.

The Imperial COVID-19 behavioural tracker

A more recent example of a mass online survey was the 'Imperial College COVID-19 behavioural tracker', organised by Imperial College, London and produced in collaboration with the surveying company yougov (Jones et al. 2020). This survey was organised to study personal feelings about the COVID-19 pandemic and assess attitudes to the measures implemented with the aim of stopping the spread of COVID-19.

Participants from 29 countries were surveyed at regular, mostly two-week, intervals from April 2020 onwards throughout the COVID-19 pandemic. They were questioned on a range of topics related to the pandemic, such as to whether they would self-isolate if told to, whether they would wear a face covering in public, the willingness to go shopping or use public transport, and the willingness to forgo social activities such as attending gatherings.

The survey was unique in that instead of simply providing a snapshot of attitudes and opinions at one specific time period, because surveying was repeated throughout the pandemic it showed how attitudes and beliefs changed over time. The regular nature of surveying meant that it was possible to assess how political and other media events influenced behaviour. For example, in the U.K. compliance to COVID-19 rules was affected when it emerged that one of the Prime Ministers most important personal advisors broke rules to travel across the country to a well known beauty spot, purportedly to test his eyesight for a longer drive.

Examination of data collected using the behavioural tracker has shown general trends in compliance in different population subgroups. For example, in my own research, those stating they had diabetes in the U.K. showed significantly higher levels of adherence to a range of protective measures than those stating no serious health condition (Walker and Lane, 2022). The willingness to self-isolate, for example, was greater in those with diabetes than for those with no health conditions. The differences remained consistent throughout the surveying period. This is of interest as those with diabetes were at a greater risk of experiencing more severe symptoms should they succumb to COVID-19. Those with diabetes thus appeared aware of the greater risk they faced and took steps to avoid infection. A different picture was seen for those with HIV/AID's though, with those with this condition showing an unexpectedly lower willingness to self-isolate than others (Lane and Walker, 2022). The use of such survey data allows such condition specific differences to be examined.

Comparison of internet and telephone questionnaires
Ghosh et al. (2008) directly compared the effectiveness of internet and telephone questionnaires in a study of disease outbreaks of norovirus and cryptosporidium in Denver, Colorado. The outbreaks studied were centred on office related luncheon parties, schools, and restaurants. Five outbreaks were investigated using internet based questionnaires, and five using telephone based questioning.

The response rate was good for both methods, being 78% to 100% for internet survey, and 60% to 100% for the telephone survey. A follow up telephone call improved response rates in both settings. The main advantage was the great saving in time the internet survey provided; telephoning took considerable time, with each conversation taking someone up to 30 minutes.

Another such comparison was conducted by Oh et al. (2010) which examined a norovirus virus outbreak following a mountain biking competition in Oregon where there were 2,273 registered riders. A survey of 95 questions was conceived. 204 of the riders were contacted to take part in the internet survey, with another 93 being contacted by telephone. There was a lower response rate for the internet survey, but in general, results were comparable.

Advantages and disadvantages

The obvious advantage of online surveying is that it offers the potential to reach a far greater range and number of people, with far greater ease, than is possible using paper based surveying. Often surveys were limited to the people one could actually question; with many academic studies centred upon college students, hospital patients or people within the locality of the survey designer. Postal surveys provided a chance to cover people over a greater geographical range, but with the added problem of cost. Physically travelling to, then asking a respondent questions, is greatly time consuming. In comparison online surveying enabled the questioning of large numbers of people, quickly and easily.

An additional advantage is that today much of the data collection and collation is automated. This means there has to be no lengthy data entry or processing. The first surveys conducted over email often did entail data processing, with the manual reading and entry of data from attached survey forms being required. However, the development of online survey platforms such as SurveyMonkey perform such tasks automatically meaning such purely online surveying is even easier.

Another advantage, which is of particular interest in the healthcare arena, is that such surveying provides a degree of anonymity (Braithwaite, 1999; Wright, 2005). This is particularly useful where the conditions being questioned about are private in nature. Sexually transmitted infections are the prime example, as there continues to remain considerable stigma related to these conditions and it is understandable that those questioned about such conditions may be reluctant to respond in face-to-face questioning. Online surveying feels, and can be made much more private and anonymous. However, this is a double edged sword. With anonymity comes the problem of knowing who is actually answering your surveys. Is the intended target audience being reached, and are respondents being honest when replying?

Online surveying can exacerbate some of the disadvantages of traditional surveying. These include self-selection bias and sampling issues. The type of people willing to respond to online questionnaires may not be representative of the population as a whole. When actually having to go out and meet respondents these factors can be controlled or managed for. Obtaining adequate response rates can be difficult and is becoming increasingly difficult. Although at one time completing an online survey was something novel, it has become routine and is now often seen as a nuisance. We have all deleted those unwanted emails asking for our opinions. Adding a financial incentive may help, but poses the additional problem of potentially affecting who answers the survey and the motives for doing so. Are people more likely to provide the answers they think are required if they believe they are being paid to do so?

REFERENCES

Braithwaite DO, Waldron VR, Finn J. Communication of social support in computer-mediated groups for people with disabilities. *Health communication*. 1999;**11**(2):123-51.

Brooks-Pollock E, Tilston N, Edmunds WJ, Eames KT. Using an online survey of healthcare-seeking behaviour to estimate the magnitude and severity of the 2009 H1N1v influenza epidemic in England. *BMC infectious diseases*. 2011;**11**(1):1-8.

Chester TL, Taylor M, Sandhu J, Forsting S, Ellis A, Stirling R, Galanis E. Use of a web forum and an online questionnaire in the detection and investigation of an outbreak. *Online journal of public health informatics*. 2011;**3**(1).

de Jong B, Ancker C. Web-based questionnaires - a tool used in a Campylobacter outbreak investigation in Stockholm, Sweden, October 2007. *Eurosurveillance.* 2008;**13**(7):pii:18847.

Evans JR, Mathur A. The value of online surveys: A look back and a look ahead. *Internet research.* 2018

Gaynor K, Katz AR, Park SY, Nataka M, Clark TA, Effler PV. Leptospirosis on Oahu: an outbreak associated with flooding of a university campus. *American journal of tropical medicine and hygiene.* 2007;**76**(5):882-885.

Ghosh TS, Patnaik JL, Alden NB, Vogt RL. Internet-versus telephone-based local outbreak investigations. *Emerging infectious diseases.* 2008;**14**(6):975-977.

Jones, SP. Imperial College COVID-19 behavioural tracker. 2020. Available at: www. imperial.ac.uk/global-health-innovation/what-we-do/our-response-to-covid-19/covid-19-behaviour-tracker/

Lane H, Walker MD. Willingness to self-isolate by those with HIV. *International journal of STD and AIDS.* 2022:09564624221096008.

Malone JL, Madjid M, Casscells SW. Telephone survey to assess influenza-like illness, United States, 2006. *Emerging infectious diseases.* 2008;**14**:129-135.

Oh JY, Bancroft JE, Cunningham MC, Keene WE, Lyss SB, Cieslak PR, Hedberg K. Comparison of survey methods in norovirus outbreak investigation, Oregon, USA, 2009. *Emerging infectious diseases.* 2010;**16**(11):1773-6.

Sugiura H, Ohkusa Y, Akahane M, Sugahara T, Okabe N, Imamura T. Construction of syndromic surveillance using a web-based daily questionnaire for health and its application at the G8 Hokkaido Toyako Summit meeting. *Epidemiology and infection.* 2010;**138**(10):1493-1502.

SurveyMonkey. SurveyMonkey User Manual. 2023. Available at:
https://s3.amazonaws.com/SurveyMonkeyFiles/UserManual.pdf

Vandendijck Y, Faes C, Hens N. Eight years of the Great Influenza Survey to monitor influenza-like illness in Flanders. *Plos one.* 2013;**8**(5):e64156.

Walker MD, Lane H. Are those with diabetes more willing to adhere to COVID-19 guidance?. *Practical diabetes.* 2022;**39**(5):23-8c.

Wright KB. Researching internet-based populations: Advantages and disadvantages of online survey research, online questionnaire authoring software packages, and web survey services. *Journal of computer-mediated communication.* 2005;**10**(3):JCMC1034.

10

REMOTE SENSING

I'm the most recognized and loved man that ever lived cuz there weren't
no satellites when Jesus and Moses were around, so people
far away in the villages didn't know about them.

Muhammad Ali.

Imagine you were a researcher investigating the environmental factors influencing the abundance and distribution of the mosquitoes which transmit malaria. The data you require might include environmental temperature, the type of vegetation present in the area you are studying, and the amount and extent of standing water such as pools or swamps. Until relatively recently, obtaining this data would probably involve organizing fieldwork into a location where the disease vector occurred. This would likely involve travel to remote areas, where transportation and communication were limited. This would be an expensive and lengthy process. Would it not be better if you could simply sit in your office, or even in the comfort of your own home, and simply download the environmental data you needed without having to go to the trouble of collecting it yourself?

Remote sensing is the collection of data without actually having to be in the location it originates from (Campbell and Wynne, 2019). It is obtaining data without making physical contact with it. The use of remote sensing technologies have become widespread in subject areas as diverse as ecology, meteorology and geography. One of the sciences which was a prime driver in the development of remote sensing technologies was oceanography, which is the science of studying the oceans. This is understandable given the difficulties of studying something the size and depth of the oceans. The U.S. National Ocean Service define remote sensing as:

> the science of obtaining information about objects or areas from a distance, typically from aircraft or satellites.
>
> (NOAA, 2021).

For a remote sensing system to function a number of components need to be in place. Firstly, you need devices or sensors capable of recording some features from a remote distance. Secondly, you need some method for this information to be sent to some data collection point. Thirdly, the ability to analyse data is required in order to interpret the data obtained.

109

Remote sensors

Remote sensors are devices which measure radiation emitted or reflected from objects. They can detect particular wavelengths of the electromagnetic spectrum. Two main forms are recognized. 'Passive' systems detect radiation which is reflected naturally from objects. In 'active' systems the sensors themselves actually emit long wavelength signals, which are then detected by the sensor when they are reflected back from the object of interest. They are recognised as they return. The output from remote sensors is often represented as two dimensional squares which relate to actual features on the ground. However, the type of data collected varies. Often a variety of data processing is required before images can be related to meaningful features on the ground. More detailed technical texts should be referred to for information on this. Remote sensors are capable of recording such physical features as vegetation, topography, and various meteorological variables such as ground temperature.

Perhaps the most basic form of remote sensing is aerial photography. A camera merely collects the light reflected from objects to produce an image. Cline (1970) was one of the first to highlight the potential of both aerial photography and remote sensing in disease science. However, today more conventionally the term remote sensing is used in reference to more complex devices, which are attached to aircraft or satellites, and where the images obtained require some processing before they are able to be used for research purposes.

The era of remote sensing can be said to have begun with the launch of the U.S. Meteorological Satellite TIROS-1 (Television Infrared Observation Satellite) in 1960. Herbreteau et al. (2007) reviewed the use of remote sensing data in epidemiological studies from 1970 to 2004, finding that most examined various parasitic conditions (59% of the studies examined). Favoured conditions of study were schistosomiasis (16%) and malaria (16%). The authors noted that it was mostly used for diseases whose distribution were heavily influenced by environmental factors.

Satellites providing remote sensing data

Landsat

Some of first remote sensing satellites were those of the Landsat program. These have been obtaining satellite images since the early 1970's. Often referred to in the singular, actually these are a series of satellites. This was a collaboration between NASA and the U.S. Geological Service. Satellites were launched in 1972, and were later renamed as Landsat in 1975. The current version, known as Landsat 9, have been operation since 2021. These satellites are mainly used to determine surface vegetation cover.

European Space Agency and Sentinel

Evolving from previous programs, the Copernicus project began in 2014 as the European Union project for world and environmental mapping. The program is made up principally of a series of Sentinel missions, each one aimed at improving land imagery in different ways. The purpose of Sentinel 1 was at obtaining radar imagery. Satellite 1A was launched in 2014 and satellite 1B in 2016. Sentinel 2 satellites which provide the capability of detailed optical imagery of land vegetation were launched in 2015 and 2017. A range of further Sentinel programs allowing detailed temperature measurement are in the process of development.

Satellites providing data of use for epidemiological purposes:

Satellite	Spatial Resolution
NOAA-AVHRR	1.1km
MODIS	1 km, 500 m, 250 m
Landsat TM/ETM+	30 m, 60 m
METEOSAT	8 km
GTOPO30	30 sec (ca. 1 km)

Data processing and analysis

As mentioned above, the data obtained from such satellites requires some processing before being of any use. This is a somewhat complex process. Most users of such data are simply concerned with obtaining usable data they can analyse themselves.

The developments in remote sensing go hand-in-hand with those in Geographical Information Systems which were described in Chapter 2. The development of various GIS programs, such as ArcView and MapInfo, allowed individual scientists to analyse the data obtained from remote sensing.

How can remote sensing data be used to monitor disease?

Environmental factors frequently influence the occurrence of disease. The temperature, humidity, and topography of an area can all affect the chances of a disease pathogen persisting in the environment. For example, rotavirus is more likely to be transmitted in cold weather than warm (Atchison et al. 2010). Another example is that the capability of bacteria such as *Escherichia coli* to persist in the environment depends on the temperature and its variability (Jang et al. 2017).

That environmental factors influence where disease occurs is maybe most obviously the case for those conditions which are vector-borne. The vectors transmitting the pathogen often have distinct climatic and environmental preferences which influence where and when they are abundant. The activity of ticks, the vectors of Lyme disease and a range of other pathogens, is influenced by temperature and humidity (Perret et al. 2000). The mosquito vectors of malaria are likewise influenced by climatic conditions, with climate change likely to influence future distributions of these parasites (Caminade et al. 2019). Remote sensing and associated GIS technology has proved most useful for studying those conditions where a link between environmental factors and disease is most apparent.

Therefore, a basic task that remotely sensed data can be used for, is in determining the climatic status of different geographical areas, and then using what is known about the requirements of a vector or disease to determine where the condition is likely to occur or be most abundant. In conjunction with data on human population levels it is even possible to extrapolate using this information in order to estimate the number of people potentially affected by the condition. Such information is of importance in determining where medical resources should be allocated.

However, such data can also be used if it is known where a disease is prevalent, to infer the climatic conditions determining its occurrence.

EXAMPLES OF REMOTE SENSING FOR DISEASE SURVEILLANCE

It is impossible to provide a comprehensive list of conditions or studies using remote sensing data. Here is a selection of some prominent or interesting studies using such data.

Predicting where Schistosomiasis occurs

Schistosomiasis is a parasitic disease caused by infection with Trematode worms from the *Schistosoma* genus (WHO, 2023). Adult worms live in human blood vessels and produce eggs, these are released into freshwater in excreta (WHO, 2023). Larvae hatch from the eggs, which then infect freshwater snails, which are a key intermediate host. Once within snails the parasites start releasing free swimming larvae into the water. People become infected when they come into contact with these larvae; they penetrate the skin and settle in the blood vessels. Schistosomiasis occurs in tropical and subtropical areas, and is reported from 78 countries. It is a major cause of long term illness, resulting in educational and economic deprivation.

Ecological factors are important in determining where the Trematode parasites which cause Schistosomiasis will occur. The environmental temperature influences the distribution of the snails that are the intermediate hosts. The snails occur only where temperatures are between 16 and 40 centigrade. Additionally, rainfall determines the extent of freshwater available for them to live in. Remote sensing offers a method to collect data on these variables. The locations where this condition occurs are often remote, rural, and economically deprived, meaning collecting climatic and weather data using traditional methods is often not possible.

Thus, remote sensing data began being used to understand the distribution of this condition as soon as data from such sources started to became available. The first studies were those of Cross and Bailey (1984) and Cross et al. (1984). These used data from the Landsat 5 Thematic Mapper (TM). They used weather parameters to map the potential occurrence of Schistosomiasis in the Philippines and the Caribbean.

Later studies looked at more detailed aspects of climate which could be influencing distribution. Malone et al. (1994) used data from the National Oceanic and Atmospheric Administration-Advanced Very High Resolution Radiometer (NOAA-AVHRR) and found that the difference in temperatures between day and night was important in potentially determining Schistosomiasis occurrence. Simoonga et al. (2009) reviewed these and other studies, as did another review by Walz et al. (2015).

Soil-transmitted helminths

Another excellent example where remote sensing data has proved useful in better understanding disease is provided by research on soil-transmitted helminths. This is the catch-all term to denote a number of parasitic infestations that humans can harbour, including roundworms *Ascaris lumbricoides*, hookworms *Necator americanus* and *Ancylostoma duodenale*, and whipworms *Trichuris trichiura*. Humans become infested with these parasites through close contact with contaminated soil. Infestation can occur either through ingestion of contaminated soil or vegetation, as is the case with roundworms. Or in the case of hookworms, infestation can occur directly through contact of the skin. These parasites are major problems in tropical areas of the globe.

Environmental parameters greatly influence the distribution of soil-transmitted helminths, with parasite presence and abundance being influenced by soil moisture, temperature, and humidity. The work of Brooker et al. (2006) emphasized that study of these environmental factors can be used to make predictions as to where such parasites will pose problems. This work also outlined how the use of remote sensing data and GIS can be used in the study of these parasites.

Many researchers have gone on to use these technologies in their own local regions. A good example where remote sensing data has been used to provide useful knowledge at the local level is demonstrated the study by Yaro et al. (2021). This used remote sensing data to produce likely abundance maps for soil-transmitted helminths for the Kogi East area of North-Central Nigeria. This study illustrates excellently how advances in technology can be used to produce information that is of importance in determining local health priorities and in potentially helping optimize resource allocation. Such studies often do not gain the recognition they deserve, but are vital.

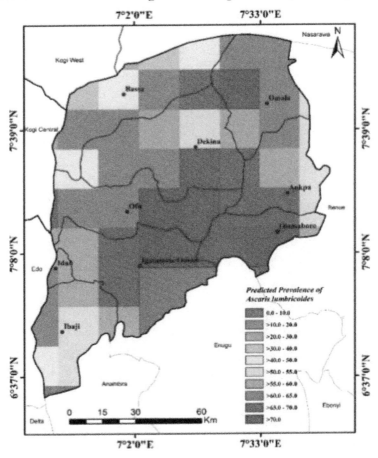

An example of how remote sensing data can help understand disease spatial distribution: Yaro et al. (2021) used remote sensing data to predict high risk areas for *A. lumbricoides* across the central part of Kogi East, Nigeria. Thank you to Clement Ameh Yaro of the Department of Animal and Environmental Biology, University of Uyo, Uyo, Akwa Ibom State, Nigeria, for permission to use.

113

Other selected examples:

Study	Details
Boone et al. (2000)	Trapped deer mice in the Walker River Basin area of Nevada/California and tested for Sin Nombre Virus. Then used remote sensed data to determine vegetation types. They could use the data to predict potential serological status of Deer Mice in new areas.
Robinson et al. (1997)	Used climatic and vegetation data to study habitat suitability of the tsetse fly *Glossina spp.*, the vector of sleeping sickness.
Sewe et al. (2017)	Used environmental data obtained from remote sensing sources to model seasonal malaria and forecast future cases. Used a type of regression known as generalized additive modeling.

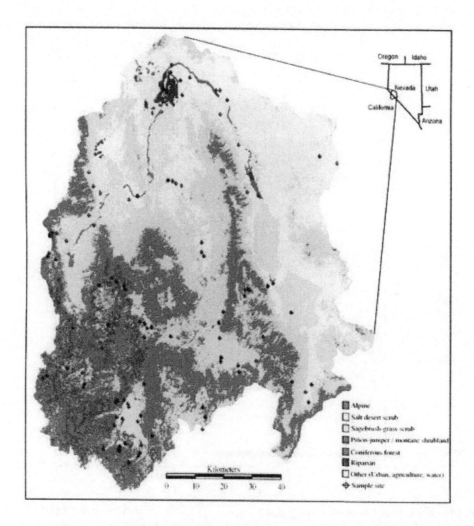

Map produced using satellite data showing vegetation types in an area of Nevada/California, which was used to study presence of Sin Nombre virus in Deer Mice. Taken from Boone et al. (2000). Please see references for citation.

Cholera

Cholera is a intestinal disease caused by infection with the bacteria *Vibrio cholerae*. It is is transmitted in water. In the Western world we think of cholera as a disease of the past; it evokes images of Victorian slums. However, in the lesser developed areas of the globe it remains a major health concern. Lobitz et al. (2000) used data obtained from remote sensing to investigate the link between cholera and climate. They obtained data on the weekly number of cholera cases occurring between 1980 and 1995. Comparing with climatic data obtained from remote sensing sources, they found a strong association with sea surface temperature.

Tsetse flies; the vector of African trypanosomiasis

Rogers and Randolf (1991) found that tsetse fly abundance in the Ivory Coast was correlated with meteorological data obtained from satellites. More recently Lord et al. (2018) used spatial data from remotely sensed sources to predict tsetse fly abundance in the Serengeti. The abundance of different *Glossina* species in different habitats was assessed through sampling, then using data relating to the landscape structure fly abundance could be extrapolated for the wider area.

Malaria

Malaria has proved an ideal candidate for remote sensing studies because the environmental parameters and vegetation preferences of the mosquito vector can be studied with such data (Rogers et al. 2002). Some examples of such studies utilizing remotely sensed data include Beck et al. (1998), who used satellite based data to identify which villages in the Southern Chiapas area of Mexico were at high or low malaria transmission risk depending on the different landscape elements in the local areas. They used landscape information to determine *Anopheles* abundance.

As described in Chapter 2, the Malaria Atlas Project provides free and easy accessible geographic information relating to malaria. Data on local, regional and national trends in malaria is provided, such as the known distributions of the *Plasmodium vivax* and *Plasmodium falciparum* parasites. The project is led by Prof. Peter Gething at Curtin University, Perth, Australia. The project provides country map profiles which are used for the WHO's annual World Malaria Report.

Advantages and disadvantages

The obvious advantages of data obtained through remote sensing are cost and ease. Obviously, some of the technologies involved are very expensive. For example, the cost of simply putting a satellite into space is extraordinarily expensive. However, the amount of data that can be collected, the range of coverage offered, and the number of potential uses such data has, means that such projects easily become cost effective. The cost and practicality of obtaining comparative data using conventional techniques for areas of the developing world would be far more costly, prohibitively so. Once the initial costs and difficulties and setting up systems are overcome remote data becomes comparatively cheap.

Developments in remote sensing have gone hand in hand with other technological developments such as the internet and Geographic Information Systems. Once obtained it is easy to share remotely sensed data. There is a growing number of people able to utilize and analyse it. Disease scientists everywhere can use such data to learn about the spatial occurrence of disease meaning that Spatial analysis is now commonplace.

But there are potential disadvantages and problems. Oversimplification may occur; the factors affecting disease occurrence may be more complex than simply being the environmental variables measured remotely by satellites. Sociological issues may influence disease occurrence, as may politics, or warfare. Remote sensing removes the incentive for more localized study which may elucidate these factors. Predictions about disease occurrence are only as good as the baseline knowledge being used in hand with remotely sensed data to make such predictions. For example, Walz et al. (2015) identified that areas used to provide an index on which to determine prevalence of Schistosomiasis can be some actual distance from the actual locations where snail hosts and freshwater they live in, is located. This could mean potentially false distribution maps could be produced.

Where next?

Increasing utilisation of machine learning methods along with remote sensing data offer the potential to make better forecasts and predictions regarding disease occurrence. Early studies using remotely sensed data often simply assessed vegetation types where disease occurs. Today more complex modelling can occur. For example, Tran et al. (2019) modelled the presence of mosquito vectors of Rift Valley fever in Senegal using meteorological data as the models input variables. As methods become refined it should be possible to forecast potential disease 'hotspots' before they even develop. Think of being able to forecast not only where flooding will occur, but where associated diseases, will be the greatest problem. For example, the rat borne condition leptospirosis occurs when flooding happens. The real time nature of remote sensing data offers the possibility of predicting where cases will begin to appear even as the rain begins to fall.

The ability to study individuals and thus ascertain individual factors influencing disease status and disease transmission should become more widespread. For example, Le Faucheur et al. (2008) studied individual walking using data obtained from Global Positioning Systems. Vazquez-Prokopec et al. (2009) Studied the potential of GPS to obtain mobility data about individuals to learn about transmission of dengue fever.

REFERENCES

Atchison CJ, Tam CC, Hajat S, Van Pelt W, Cowden JM, Lopman BA. Temperature-dependent transmission of rotavirus in Great Britain and The Netherlands. *Proceedings of the royal society B: Biological sciences.* 2010;**277**(1683):933-42.

Beck LR, Rodriguez MH, Dister SW, Rodriguez AD, Rejmankova E, Ulloa A, Meza RA, Roberts DR, Paris JF, Spanner MA. Remote sensing as a landscape epidemiologic tool to identify villages at high risk for malaria transmission. *The American journal of tropical medicine and hygiene.* 1994;**51**(3):271-80.

Boone JD, McGwire KC, Otteson EW, DeBaca RS, Kuhn EA, Villard P, Brussard PF, St Jeor SC. Remote sensing and geographic information systems: charting Sin Nombre virus infections in deer mice. *Emerging infectious diseases.* 2000;**6**(3):248.

Brooker S, Clements AC, Bundy DA. Global epidemiology, ecology and control of soil-transmitted helminth infections. *Advances in parasitology.* 2006;**62**:221-61.

Campbell JB, Wynne RH. Introduction to Remote Sensing. 5th ed. Guilford Press, New York, NY. 2011.

Caminade C, McIntyre KM, Jones AE. Impact of recent and future climate change on vector-borne diseases. *Annals of the New York academy of sciences.* 2019;**1436**:157-173.

Cline BL. New eyes for epidemiologists: aerial photography and other remote sensing techniques. *American journal of epidemiology*. 1970;**92**:85-89.

Cross ER, Bailey RC. Prediction of areas endemic for schistosomiasis through use of discriminant analysis of environmental data. *Military medicine*. 1984;**149**(1):28-30.

Cross ER, Perrine R, Sheffield C, Pazzaglia G. Predicting areas endemic for Schistosomiasis using weather variables and a Landsat Data Base. *Military medicine*. 1984;**149**(10):542-544.

Herbreteau V, Salem G, Souris M, Hugot JP, Gonzalez JP. Thirty years of use and improvement of remote sensing, applied to epidemiology: from early promises to lasting frustration. *Health and place*. 2007;**13**(2):400-3.

Jang J, Hur HG, Sadowsky MJ, Byappanahalli MN, Yan T, Ishii S. Environmental Escherichia coli: ecology and public health implications—a review. *Journal of applied microbiology*. 2017;**123**(3):570-81.

Le Faucheur A, Abraham P, Jaquinandi V, Bouyé P, Saumet JL, Noury-Desvaux B. Measurement of walking distance and speed in patients with peripheral arterial disease: a novel method using a global positioning system. *Circulation*. 2008;**117**(7):897-904.

Lobitz B, Beck L, Huq A, Wood B, Fuchs G, Faruque AS, Colwell R. Climate and infectious disease: use of remote sensing for detection of Vibrio cholerae by indirect measurement. *Proceedings of the national academy of sciences*. 2000;**97**(4):1438-43.

Lord JS, Torr SJ, Auty HK, Brock PM, Byamungu M, Hargrove JW, Morrison LJ, Mramba F, Vale GA, Stanton MC. Geostatistical models using remotely-sensed data predict savanna tsetse decline across the interface between protected and unprotected areas in Serengeti, Tanzania. *Journal of applied ecology*. 2018;**55**(4):1997-2007.

Malaria Atlas Project. 2022. Available at: https://malariaatlas.org/

Malone JB, Huh OK, Fehler DP, Wilson PA, Wilensky DE, Holmes RA, Elmagdoub AI. Temperature data from satellite imagery and the distribution of schistosomiasis in Egypt. *The American journal of tropical medicine and hygiene*. 1994;**50**(6):714-22.

National Oceanic and Atmospheric Administration (NAOO). What is remote sensing? 2021. Available at: www.oceanservice.noaa.gov/facts/remotesensing.html

Robinson T, Rogers D, Williams B. Mapping tsetse habitat suitability in the common fly belt of Southern Africa using multivariate analysis of climate and remotely sensed vegetation data. *Medical and veterinary entomology*. 1997;**11**(3):235-245.

Rogers DJ, Randolph SE, Snow RW, Hay SI. Satellite imagery in the study and forecast of malaria. *Nature*. 2002;**415**(6872):710-5.

Rogers DJ, Randolph SE. Mortality rates and population density of tsetse flies correlated with satellite imagery. *Nature*. 1991;**351**(6329):739-41.

Sewe MO, Tozan Y, Ahlm C, Rocklöv J. Using remote sensing environmental data to forecast malaria incidence at a rural district hospital in Western Kenya. *Scientific reports*. 2017;**7**(1):1-0.

Simoonga C, Utzinger J, Brooker S, Vounatsou P, Appleton CC, Stensgaard AS, Olsen A, Kristensen TK. Remote sensing, geographical information system and spatial analysis for schistosomiasis epidemiology and ecology in Africa. *Parasitology*. 2009;**136**(13):1683-93.

Tran A, Fall AG, Biteye B, Ciss M, Gimonneau G, Castets M, Seck MT, Chevalier V. Spatial modeling of mosquito vectors for Rift Valley fever virus in Northern Senegal: Integrating satellite-derived meteorological estimates in population dynamics models. *Remote sensing*. 2019;**11**(9):1024.

Vazquez-Prokopec GM, Stoddard ST, Paz-Soldan V, Morrison AC, Elder JP, Kochel TJ, Scott TW, Kitron U. Usefulness of commercially available GPS data-loggers for tracking human movement and exposure to dengue virus. *International journal of health geographics.* 2009;8(1):1-1.

Walz Y, Wegmann M, Dech S, Raso G, Utzinger J. Risk profiling of schistosomiasis using remote sensing: approaches, challenges and outlook. *Parasites and vectors.* 2015;**8**:163.

World Health Organisation (WHO). Schistosomiasis: key facts. 2023. Available at: www.who.int/news-room/fact-sheets/detail/schistosomiasis

Yaro CA, Kogi E, Luka SA, Nassan MA, Kabir J, Opara KN, Hetta HF, Batiha GE. Edaphic and climatic factors influence on the distribution of soil transmitted helminths in Kogi East, Nigeria. *Scientific reports.* 2021; **11**:8490.

11

SALES AND PRODUCT REVIEW DATA

Follow the money

Deep Throat, from the film 'All the
Presidents Men', 1976.

'Cure all diseases' was the claim made on the bottle of the quack medicine 'Microbe Killer'. This product, peddled by William Radam in 1880's America, was a useless mixture of sulphuric acid and red wine. Despite its ineffectiveness, Radam did very well from 'Microbe Killer' and gained both public and medical notoriety.

When we feel ill it is natural that we will seek out some way to alleviate our symptoms. Business people are eager to supply products to fulfil this need. In the days of 'Microbe Killer' there were no consumer protection laws. However, today the medical products market is strictly regulated. A vast array of products are available allowing self treatment. Often these are available to purchase from local chemists, or even supermarkets, and are known generally as 'over-the-counter' (OTC) products. Data relating to the sales of such products offers a useful potential source of information about how common a particular condition could be.

Modern retail

Just like every other avenue in life, retail is a field which has been revolutionized by modern computing and technology. Forget old style notebook purchase and sales ledgers. Modern logistics is complex and heavily computerized. Databases contain inventories of stock which are updated as soon as a bar code is scanned by a cashier at the till. Products can be re-ordered automatically as soon as stock levels begin to run low. The concept of 'just-in-time' is used to denote meeting customer demand as quickly as possible, without products being stored unnecessarily in warehouses. Storage is expensive and moving products into and out of warehouses creates additional labour costs. The ideal is for products to come from a supplier and end up instantly on the shelves of local branches.

Sales data and epidemiology

The potential of using sales for epidemiological purposes was realised well before the development of machine learning and personal computing. In the late 1970's the potential of using sales of cold and flu remedies to study trends in influenza cases was realized by researchers (Welliver et al.

119

1979). However, at that time systems for obtaining information in a timely manner were lacking. Much of the information required by epidemiologists was not computerized then.

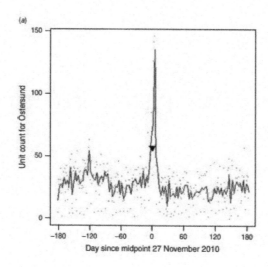

Figure from Andersson et al. (2014). This study examined the potential of a variety of data sources at detecting local outbreaks. This figure shows OTC sales of anti-diarrhoeal products from pharmacies during an outbreak of gastrointestinal illness. The study looked at the ability of different data science methods to spot disease outbreaks. Telephone data from a healthcare hotline spotted four of the four largest outbreaks; web search data spotted one, and OTC sales data spotted two.

Cryptosporidiosis in Milwaukee

A large outbreak of cryptosporidiosis occurred in Milwaukee in 1993. This bacterial infection can be contracted through contact with infected water. It results in diarrhoeal illness, which can be quite severe and last several days. Rodman et al. (1997) noted increases in the sales of anti-diarrhoeal products from local pharmacists coinciding with cases. Daily sales of such products increased from $30 to $600 during the outbreak, a 20 fold increase.

The article by Rodman also looked at the potential of sales data for epidemiology more widely. It found that that 10 U.S. states were already using some form of surveillance based upon sales data. The study identified a number of disease outbreaks where increases in sales of related products had occurred and been identified. The study also detailed the use of data from a drug distributor in New Mexico which was used by disease epidemiologists to assess potentially developing disease problems. This article helped highlight the potential of such data for syndromic surveillance.

A new impetus: spotting an anthrax bio-terrorism attack

Could you spot when an bio-terrorist anthrax attack is occurring by examining cough medicine sales? The U.S. anthrax bio-terrorism incident of 2001 was an impetus to the development of systems based upon sales data. After this attack there was much obviously much interest in being able to spot future such attacks, and data from OTC sales was one potential method. Goldenberg et al. (2002) attempted to develop a monitoring system using OTC sales of cough medicines. A problem was that the sales of drug store cough medicines vary naturally over time anyway, making it difficult to spot unusual trends or spikes. As the authors noted, this is a very noisy dataset. They broke the time series down, using cosine transformation, to try to identify relatively small changes in sales that might occur due to a small and localized release of anthrax in the community.

An anthrax attack had occurred in 1979 in Sverdlovsk, Russia. The authors attempted to simulate a similar scale event of an attack on 77 people. They then looked to see if the method they had developed could detect it. Although the system proved promising, it proved difficult to spot an attack of such a small size among a much larger population. They suggested that using a range of products might prove more effective at spotting unusual spikes in sales data that might be indicative of such an attack.

Systems for the surveillance of OTC sales often date from the early 2000's. The New York City (NYC) Department of Health and Mental Hygiene (DOHMH) started monitoring sales of cough and cold remedies to provide an indication of influenza-like-illness and of antidiarrhoeal products to indicate possible gastrointestinal illness outbreaks in 2002. They use linear regression techniques to spot changes in expected sales patterns (Das et al 2005).

Do pharmacy store sales equate to illness?
A key question before syndromic surveillance systems can be established using sales data is whether the sales of a particular product actually indicate corresponding trends in a particular ailment. Most emphasis has been on those conditions with clear severe symptoms and which are readily treatable without the need to consult medical professionals. A number of studies have thus examined influenza-like-illnesses and whether sales of 'cold' remedies can be used to provide forewarning of impending spikes. Gastrointestinal ailments are also popular for study, with symptoms such as diarrhoea being readily treatable with products such as electrolyte.

Davies and Finch (2003) examined hospital admissions for respiratory illness in the British city of Nottingham and looked to see if there was an association with sales of cold and flu products at local 'Boots' chemists stores. They also looked to see if trends corresponded to data from a national website providing information on influenza incidence; the 'Lemsip FluForecast'. They examined sales data for cough and cold remedies over three Winters, 1998/99 to 2001/2002. They found a correlation between local sales and influenza. Then they used national sales data to forecast what levels of influenza were nationally. They found that peaks in emergency admissions could be predicted two weeks beforehand using information of local OTC sales. However, this peak was somewhat expected, as it regularly occurs during Winter.

An example of a study looking at gastrointestinal illness is the work of Pivette et al. (2014). Using a database of sales from a network of French community pharmacists, they examined whether purchases of treatments for gastrointestinal complaints could be used to forecast seasonal peaks. In Europe, medical products are classed according to which symptoms they help alleviate, and the authors looked at those classes related to gastrointestinal conditions, which included antidiarrhoeal products. Sales data was compared to data on the number of cases of acute diarrhoea obtained from a sentinel network of medical practitioners.

Separately, the same authors conducted a review into the effectiveness of studies using pharmaceutical sales data (Pivette et al. 2014). This review examined 27 studies that used sales data. It found that gastroenteritis infections and acute respiratory infections were the most commonly studied ailments in such studies. This appears logical as such ailments can occur as outbreaks with large numbers of people being affected; this means clear effects on sales data should be apparent. Additionally, these ailments have rather distinct symptoms against which a number of well known and effective remedies exist. Self-care is typical for conditions such as diarrhoea, constipation, coughs and sore throats. Typically, a doctors appointment won't be made for such minor complaints. The review found that most studies compared levels of medicinal drug sales to clinical data, with 17 of the 19 studies examined finding strong correlations between the two. A number of the studies looked at found that trends in sales data preceded corresponding trends in clinical data; potentially of great use for those tasked with establishing disease surveillance systems.

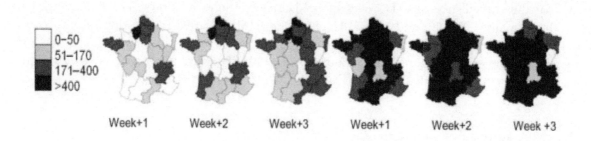

Vergu et al. (2006) used medicament sales to improve forecasting of influenza-like-illness across France. Image from Emerging Infectious Diseases, 2006; 416-21.

Finding the palette of treatments related to specific conditions

The majority of studies simply look for a correlation between sales data for a specific product, or handful of products, and a specific ailment. But increasingly common is to examine which palette of drugs best correlates with specific conditions (Magrunder, 2003). For example, Sočan et al. (2012) found that modelling was best with certain medicament types than others; mucolytics and antitussives, Medicines for Sore Throats and decongestants resulted in the best performing Poisson regression models.

Wallstrom and Hogan (2007) developed algorithms which could identify which clusters of treatment drugs were related to which medical conditions, which is potentially of great help in developing syndromic surveillance systems. Only a handful of studies have gone further and used such data for active surveillance.

Examining sales data can't always be considered to be effective, and seems to only be effective for specific conditions, at specific locations. For example, a study by Kirian and Weintraub (2010) failed to show any relationship between anti-diarrhoea product sales and related illness, and forecasting proved ineffective.

Selected studies using sales data to examine disease incidence.

Study	Details
Edge et al. (2006)	Norovirus activity and sales of OTC sales for gastrointestinal ailments showed similar patterns.
Harrison et al. (2014)	Investigated whether online restaurant reviews could be used to find disease outbreaks. Software analysed 294,000 reviews, with 893 providing indications of a food borne illness. Telephone interviewing of 27 reviewers identified three previously potential unreported outbreaks.
Hogan et al. (2003)	Studied sales of electrolyte and infectious respiratory and diarrhoea paediatric disease. There was a very high correlation between sales and the diseases studied. Sales may precede illness, but depended on year studied.
Li et al. (2005)	Studied which diagnoses correlated best with electrolyte sales
Liu et al. (2013)	Examined the relationship between pharmaceutical sales and patients attending an urgent care centre with influenza-like-illness for thirteen zip codes around the greater Pittsburgh area. Sales among the cough and cold and temperature retail categories were correlated with cases during influenza season.

Different avenues

Actual sales data is not the only commercial information source that could be used. There are other potential sources:

Product reviews: Another potential avenue for epidemiological research are product reviews on online forums. Although rather a blunt instrument, it could well be that the volume these are visited indicates possible upsurges in cases of particular illnesses.

Table reservations: In an ingenious study, Nsoesie et al. (2014) examined whether there was a relationship between table reservations and influenza. The authors postulated that as influenza increasingly circulated in a population, then restaurant table availability would increase. This would be because people felt ill or simply 'off' and thus would not feel like going out to dinner.

The authors obtained data on table reservations covering 10 regions of the U.S. and Mexico from an online restaurant portal 'OpenTable'. They then examined whether the data correlated with data from Google Flu Trends and official state level influenza reports. They found that there were potentially correlations at the local level. Although limited, the results suggest such data could be used to provide a rough and ready early indication of when influenza rates were rising.

Prescription or Medicaid data: Another potential source of data are examining records of when treatment has been prescribed. The advantage of such data is that it is already digitized, and often already present in the health care system, meaning accessing it should be easier than that of sales data from commercial enterprises. Chen et al. (2005) described how treatment of cases of pertussis, plus prophylactic treatment of contacts, resulted in a clear signal above baseline levels in Medicaid data on prescriptions for macrolide antibiotics. This suggested that such data could be used in future outbreak detection.

Advantages and disadvantages

A first advantage is that the sales data for some specific drugs is likely to correspond to the incidence of particular specific complaints. For example, there is a good chance that purchases of anti-diarrhoeal products will be related to gastrointestinal complaints, as shown by a number of studies . However, a number of complaints share similar symptoms, and some products may be used to treat a range of conditions. One only has to think of aspirin or paracetamol, which have a wide range of uses; disentangling whether sales of these products is related to any one condition will be difficult.

Sales data is likely to be best for syndromic surveillance where case numbers of a condition are high, meaning that 'noise' caused by purchases for other reasons become less important. Influenza would be the best example, as large numbers of people suffer from this condition each year, thus sales data aimed at alleviating its symptoms are likely to reflect influenza incidence well.

Sales data offers other advantages. In developed countries, the network of local pharmacies is well developed. As digital management improves, obtaining sales data at an increasingly local scale should become more and more feasible. Such data offers the opportunity to examine patterns in infectious diseases at a local scale. Spikes in the purchases of products should be more readily apparent locally.

Disadvantages include the obvious noise in such data, as was pointed our in the study by Andersson et al. (2014). Anther problem is that the statistical methods used to detect anomalies can be complex, as shown in the study by Que and Tsui (2012) who compared algorithms using sales data on thermometer sales. People may purchase products without really requiring them, or buy them for reasons other than their intended purpose. The general public is becoming increasingly health aware; reports of health issues in the media and press may result in spikes in purchases of corresponding treatments, without their actually being an increase in cases. During the initial COVID-19 pandemic sales of paracetamol spiked, as people stocked up 'just in case'.

Another problem is being able to process data quickly enough. Local pharmacy networks may be linked administratively to local health care systems, meaning sales data might reach local public health officials quickly. But where private companies are involved there may be delays in public health officials obtaining such data. Sales data may be considered commercially sensitive, so there may be reluctance from companies to release it; requiring the need for some form of indexing so that underlying patterns remain, but the actual amount of turnover remains unknown.

What next?

Commerce is being increasingly conducted online, with retailers such as Amazon gaining global dominance. This offers new opportunities for the epidemiologist wanting to use sales data for syndromic surveillance. The possibility of obtaining information on patterns in online searching for products designed for certain conditions remains a possibility, thus providing information before sales are even made. Those retailing through Amazon can receive detailed data on when products are sold and where. Although there are potential data protection issues here, should those interested in public health be able to obtain similar data there is great promise here.

In an interesting twist, Mackay et al. (2020) examined sales of questionable products related to the COVID-19 pandemic. This shows the opportunistic nature of people and there readiness to try to make money whenever they can. The authors analysed Tweets and other sources for sales pitches for such products, noting a number of waves of COVID-19 products. In the first wave were herbal and fake cures, and in the second PPE and testing kits.

REFERENCES

Andersson T, Bjelkmar P, Hulth A, Lindh J, Stenmark S, Widerström M. Syndromic surveillance for local outbreak detection and awareness: evaluating outbreak signals of acute gastroenteritis in telephone triage, web-based queries and over-the-counter pharmacy sales. *Epidemiology and infection.* 2014;**142**(2):303-13.

Chen JH, Schmit K, Chang H, Herlihy E, Miller J, Smith P. Use of Medicaid prescription data for syndromic surveillance. *MMWR Morbidity and mortality weekly report.* 2005:**31**.

Das D, Metzger K, Heffernan R, Balter S, Weiss D, Mostashari F. Monitoring over-the-counter medication sales for early detection of disease outbreaks—New York City. *MMWR Morbidity and mortality weekly report.* 2005;**54**(Suppl):41-6.

Davies GR, Finch RG. Sales of over-the-counter remedies as an early warning system for Winter bed crises. *Clinical microbiology and infection.* 2003;**9**:858-863.

Edge VL, Pollari F, King L, Michel P, McEwen SA, Wilson JB, Jerrett M, Sockett PN, Martin SW. Syndromic surveillance of norovirus using over the counter sales of medications related to gastrointestinal illness. *Canadian journal of infectious diseases and medical microbiology.* 2006;**17**(4):235-41.

Goldenberg A, Shmueli G, Caruana RA, Fienberg SE. Early statistical detection of anthrax outbreaks by tracking over-the-counter medication sales. *Proceedings of the national academy of science USA.* 2002;**99**(8):5237-40.

Harrison C, Jorder M, Stern H, Stavinsky F, Reddy V, Hanson H, Waechter H, Lowe L, Gravano L, Balter S. Using online reviews by restaurant patrons to identify unreported cases of foodborne illness—New York City, 2012–2013. *MMWR Morbidity and mortality weekly report.* 2014;**63**(20):441.

Hogan WR, Tsui FC, Ivanov O, Gesteland PH, Grannis S, Overhage JM, Robinson JM, Wagner MM. Detection of pediatric respiratory and diarrheal outbreaks from sales of over-the-counter electrolyte products. *Journal of the American medical informatics association.* 2003;**10**(6):555-62.

Kirian ML, Weintraub JM. Prediction of gastrointestinal disease with over-the-counter diarrheal remedy sales records in the San Francisco Bay Area. *BMC medical informatics and decision making.* 2010;**10**(1):1-9.

Li R, Wallstrom GL, Hogan WR. A multivariate procedure for identifying correlations between diagnoses and over-the-counter products from historical datasets. In: AMIA Annual Symposium Proceedings 2005 (Vol. 2005, p. 450). American Medical Informatics Association.

Liu TY, Sanders JL, Tsui FC, Espino JU, Dato VM, Suyama J. Association of over-the-counter pharmaceutical sales with influenza-like-illnesses to patient volume in an urgent care setting. *Plos one.* 2013;**8**(3):e59273.

Mackey TK, Li J, Purushothaman V, Nali M, Shah N, Bardier C, Cai M, Liang B. Big data, natural language processing, and deep learning to detect and characterize illicit COVID-19 product sales: Infoveillance study on Twitter and Instagram. *JMIR public health and surveillance.* 2020;**6**(3):e20794.

Magruder S. Evaluation of over-the-counter pharmaceutical sales as a possible early warning indicator of human disease. *Johns Hopkins University APL Technical Digest.* 2003;**24**(4):349-53.

Nsoesie E, Buckeridge D, Brownstein J. Guess Who's Not Coming to Dinner? Evaluating Online Restaurant Reservations for Disease Surveillance. *Journal of medical internet research.* 2014;**16**.

Pivette M, Mueller JE, Crepey P, Bar-Hen A. Surveillance of gastrointestinal disease in France using drug sales data. *Epidemics.* 2014;**8**:1-8.

Pivette M, Mueller JE, Crépey P, Bar-Hen A. Drug sales data analysis for outbreak detection of infectious diseases: a systematic literature review. *BMC infectious diseases.* 2014;**14**(1):1-4.

Que J, Tsui FC. Spatial and temporal algorithm evaluation for detecting over-the-counter thermometer sale increases during 2009 H1N1 pandemic. *Online journal of public health informatics.* 2012;**4**(1).

Rodman JS, Frost F, Davis-Burchat L, Fraser D. Pharmaceutical sales--a method of disease surveillance?. *Journal of environmental health.*1997;**60**(4):8.

Sočan M, Erčulj V, Lajovic J. Early detection of influenza-like illness through medication sales. *Central European journal of public health.* 2012;**20**(2):156-62.

Vergu E, Grais RF, Sarter H, Fagot JP, Lambert B, Valleron AJ, Flahault A. Medication sales and syndromic surveillance, France. *Emerging infectious diseases.* 2006;**12**(3):416.

Wallstrom GL, Hogan WR. Unsupervised clustering of over-the-counter healthcare products into product categories. *Journal of biomedical informatics.* 2007;**40**(6):642-8.

Welliver RC, Cherry JD, Boyer KM, Deseda-Tous JE, Krause PJ, Dudley JP, Murray RA, Wingert W, Champion JG, Freeman G. Sales of nonprescription cold remedies: a unique method of influenza surveillance. *Pediatric research.* 1979;**13**(9):1015-7.

12

SCHOOL ATTENDANCE DATA

We don't need no education.

The Who, British Band.

Can children be used as disease sentinels? All children have to, or should be, receiving an education. For the vast majority of children in the developed world this normally entails attending a formal educational institute, such as a nursery or school, typically on a daily basis. Attendance is traditionally recorded through the taking of registers kept on a daily basis. Sometimes attendance at individual lessons is recorded. Increasingly this is becoming a digital process, often with students scanning bar coded identity cards.

Records relating to school attendance are of interest to the disease epidemiologist because children are embedded in society, belonging to families and interacting widely in society. Often a child's level of social interaction is greater than many adults, particularly elderly ones. Children interact with other children of their own and different ages, with siblings, with their parents, and often with their grandparents. As every parent knows, if any bug is doing the rounds, it is children who get it first! Can we use these facts to study disease occurrence and use children to provide a forewarning of forthcoming outbreaks?

Influenza and school absenteeism
Examination of school attendance data to study disease precedes the digital age with studies existing from the 1980's onwards. A number of studies have utilized school attendance data to examine whether levels of absenteeism are related to influenza. Although the methods used in each study vary, generally patterns in absenteeism are studied and whether these correspond to patterns seen in officially recorded case numbers of influenza.

One example is Williams et al. (2013) who examined school attendance during the H1N1 influenza pandemic of 2009. Children were thought to be disproportionately greatly affected. The authors examined absences from schools in Denver, Colorado. They compared these to the numbers of confirmed cases in hospitals. Data running from Kindergarten through to grade 12 was used. There was little correlation between confirmed hospital cases of influenza and school absenteeism. However, the cause of absenteeism was not listed, and could have been due to something else other than influenza. But there was a notable positive correlation between confirmed cases and visits to school health offices specifically for influenza-like-illness. The best correlation was found when school absences were lagged by one week, effectively showing that rises in illness in schools occurred before corresponding changes in confirmed case data, thus showing the promise of this data at anticipating future incidence.

In another study produced during this period, school nurses in Maryland were asked to complete a daily online questionnaire about school illness and absenteeism (Crawford et al. 2011). They were questioned as to the percentage of absenteeism within their schools, and the number of visits to the school health rooms by students with influenza like symptoms. The study comprised 80 schools for those aged between five and 12 years of age. Data was compared to an established syndromic surveillance system, ESSENCE, which collates data from hospital emergency attendances and uses them to provide an indication of future potential disease outbreaks. The results found that the number of visits to health rooms for influenza like symptoms mirrored data from emergency hospitals, with a high correlation between the two being found. The relationship between absenteeism and ESSENCE data, was however not as strong, with no notable correlation being found.

The study by Ma et al. (2014) compared different syndromic systems over four influenza seasons, one of which was based on school absenteeism. Data was obtained from a private company managing attendance data for 500 both elementary and high schools in Sweden. The data used did not consider the reason for absence, and gave the proportion of absent students out of the total number of students included. The correlation between the school absence data and that from sentinel clinicians and laboratory confirmed cases was low. This maybe shows that more specific data on the specific reasons for school absences is needed, or that data for discrete age ranges may be more effective and showing correlations.

A number of studies have been conducted in the U.K. Zhao et al. (2007) highlighted that influenza outbreaks occurring in English and Welsh schools in 2006 and 2007 were not picked up by the surveillance systems being used then, and suggested implementing school based surveillance based on absence data. Aldridge et al (2016) described a study which combined disease surveillance with public engagement with science. Through an educational program students in the schools where data was collected learnt about the data itself and practised using it.

Measuring absenteeism
Studies vary in how they measure absenteeism. This has been found to affect the strength of association with the metric of influenza being used. For example, Schmidt et al. (2010) examined attendance data from six primary school in East London. The authors found that the peaks in the absence prevalence correlated better with lab confirmed cases of influenza than did data showing the incidence of absence.

Another common practice is to study when absence hits certain thresholds and use that as a predictor of an outbreak. This could be either when a certain percentage of students are absent due to illness of all kinds, or specifically due to influenza-like-illness. This is simpler than using complex mathematical procedures. Kom Mogto et al (2012) studying school absenteeism in Quebec elementary and secondary schools during the 2009 H1N1 pandemic used a 10% threshold, and found good correlations with lab confirmed cases and hospitalization levels in children. However, the authors could not determine whether absences preceded confirmed cases. Absenteeism rates were greater for primary age children than secondary, suggesting that different thresholds of reporting might be appropriate for different age ranges. Other studies using thresholds in a similar manner include Sasaki et al (2009) which used the 10% threshold, and Lenaway and Ambler (1995) which used a 7.5% threshold. Some studies such as Cheng et al. (2012) examine the peak in absenteeism, while others have used mean absenteeism instead.

Differences in school attendance from one period to another might not be obvious. There are a great number of days when children do go to school and thus are not absent, well hopefully. So the number of days absent will not be great. Song et al. (2018) worked around this problem by using zero inflated Poisson modelling. First they fitted data in one year to a Poisson model, then predicted events for a second year, comparing the expected with the observed pattern of absence. This makes any difference more apparent.

The head louse and school attendance

The wonderfully elegant parasite the head louse, dwells among the hair follicles of the head where it lays its 'nit' eggs. They are not a serious problem, although they can cause irritation and some slight skin complaints. However, infestation is considered unpleasant and socially undesirable. Children, particularly those in younger age ranges are particularly prone to becoming infested. They lack awareness of personal space, and frequent head bumping and boisterous physical play promote transmission.

Educational attendance was greatly affected during the COVID-19 year of 2020. Home schooling was implemented for much of the year, and even continued into the Spring of 2021. Given that the head louse relies so much on school age contact for transmission, did its incidence decline during this period?

Google Trends data would appear to suggest so, with internet searching on the head louse dropping by over 40% from pre-pandemic level. Walker and Sulyok (2023) examined whether internet searching on the head louse was related to school attendance data, but found no strong correlation between the two. However, that social distancing restrictions had an effect on internet searching on head lice was clear. There were notable reductions.

Cryptosporidiosis and school absence data

Few studies exist which examine non-influenza-like-illnesses and the relationship with school attendance One such study is that by Proctor et al. (1998). A cryptosporidiosis outbreak occurred in Milwaukee in March and April 1993. The authors collected data from a range of surveillance sources, including data from nursing homes, water treatment plants, and school absence logs. They then assessed the potential of each at providing forewarning of an outbreak. A peak in school absences occurred on the 6th of April, about a week prior to a corresponding peak seen in clinical data which occurred on the 12th of April. The peak in school data was in line with peaks seen in nursing home data and Emergency Department data, but later than indications available from water treatment facilities. A key problem was the time it took for data to become available; 64 days; making this the slowest form of surveillance in terms of data availability.

Example studies examining school attendance or absence data and disease occurrence

Study	Condition examined	Method	Statistical Method	Finding
Aldridge et al. (2016)	Influenza	27 schools provided data from 2011 to 2013. Looked at daily school absence and compared with incidence of ILI recorded by Royal College of General Practitioners	Linear regression	Strong association between absence and Royal College of General Practise sentinel data on ILI.
Besculides et al. (2005)	Influenza	Examined NYC Department of Education attendance data.	Used CuSum method to find periods with unusual attendance patterns.	Found that periods of low attendance were related to peak influenza season.
Bollaerts et al. (2010)	Influenza	Daily absence data for workers and schools was compared to GP sentinel data on ILI in Belgium.	Percentage absence data used and scatter plotted using smoothing.	Peaks in absenteeism occurred prior to peaks in ILI cases.
Cheng et al. (2012)	Influenza	Illustrated electronic automatic recording of school absences.	Compared peaks from difference methods.	Peaks in school absences coincided with peaks in sentinel GP and lab confirmed cases.
Mann et al. (2011)	Influenza-like-illness	Miama Dade County, Florida.	Assessment of a syndromic surveillance system identifying clusters of ILI from automatically recorded absenteeism data.	Clusters of ILI/H1N1 were identified showing the effectiveness of the system.
Kom Mogto et al. (2012)	Influenza	Schools in Quebec electronically reported when absence due to ILI exceeded 10%.		Correlation with lab confirmed cases and hospitalisation in infants was high.
Proctor et al. (1998)	Cryptosporidiosis	School absence data from Milwaukee schools following an outbreak in 1993.	Compared absence data at providing forewarning with other surveillance methods.	Peaks in school absence data were apparent and occurred prior to indicators obtained from clinical data, but the length of time in getting data was long.
Suzue et al. (2012)	Influenza	Describes establishment of a School Absence Reporting System for Infectious Diseases in Japan.		School data proved more sensitive than data from national surveillance.

ILI = influenza-like-illness

Advantages

One advantage of using school absence data is that changes in school attendance are likely to occur immediately once an illness begins to circulate in the wider population; children get ill first. They are effectively the canaries in the mine providing a forewarning of problems that might develop in the wider population. Children are likely to be removed from school when 'poorly', meaning potential changes in school attendance occur as soon as illness starts to circulate (Bollaerts et al. 2010).

A second advantage is that this type of surveillance is fairly generic and broad based (Bollaerts et al. 2010). We don't know what the underlying cause of the next disease outbreak will be, nor which symptoms we need to look out for. School absence data provides a general bell-weather that could indicate a variety of conditions.

Other potential benefits include that this type of data should be easily available and cheap. It is being collected anyway. With increasing digitization, it should be easily possible to establish automatic monitoring procedures, or the ready transfer of data between educational institutes and health care professionals.

Problems and disadvantages

One problem with school based syndromic surveillance is that it can be difficult to obtain the required data quickly enough. Karo et al. (2011) found that peaks in weekly school absence coincided with other forms of syndromic surveillance during the H1N1 influenza pandemic, and noted that availability of daily data might have shown rises in absenteeism earlier. Kom Mogto et al. (2012) also were only able to obtain data on a weekly basis. The data is collected by schools, or education officials, and the transfer of this to health officials can take time. The transfer of such files can occur automatically, but as Mann et al. (2011) noted, it is still often the case that such absenteeism is recorded manually. This can delay the process, as such paper records need to be transferred into an electronic format. Procedures need to be put into place to ensure that data can be obtained on a daily basis and be available to health officials immediately.

However, perhaps the main problem limiting the use of school attendance data is that although absence might be recorded and a cause given, this might not actually reflect the true reason for the absence. It is often easier for parents to cite illness as the reason for absence, especially when the true reason would not be deemed sufficient to permit absence. It could well be the case that parents knowing that a 'bug' is going around, use this as the reason to account for a school absence, thus potentially amplifying the effect. As Besculides et al. (2005) notes, such data is 'noisy', meaning that spikes and anomalies may not be related to actual disease outbreaks. Although educational facilities can be large in size, even the largest schools will only number in the hundreds of pupils, meaning that the volume of potential people from who data can be collected from may not be large enough to determine underlying population trends. Pooling of data over school areas may be required. A number of studies described here, examined the period of the H1N1 'swine flu' influenza outbreak (e.g. Mann et al. 2011); the relationship between school absence and clinical data could have been unusually strong in this period.

131

Other potential problems include:

- **Data availability:** Data is only available when children are at school. There are large periods of the year which are school holidays. For those in the northern hemisphere two to three weeks is typically taken for holidays in December; exactly at that the time of year when epidemiologists would most like such data.

- **Data reliability:** Absence from school does not necessarily mean illness. For example, package holidays are considerably cheaper when taken in term time, and many parents feign illness in their children to take advantage.

- **A blunt tool:** Typically the reason for illness or absence is not recorded. Thus, the data on absences relates to absences caused by all illnesses and conditions circulating at that time. Trying to entangle the influence of one specific condition among the rest is thus difficult.

- **Are children falling ill first?** The assumption is often made that children fall ill before other age groups. But this may not be the case. Children typically tend not to experience severe illness, and for some illnesses may even be asymptomatic.

- **Studies are limited:** A limitation of studies is that most are limited over time, examining usually a single year, or at most two years. A large number examined the period of the H1N1 influenza pandemic, which could well be an unusual period.

Where next?

School attendance data has much promise. But more examination is needed as to whether it provides reliable year-on-year surveillance. The best methods of interpreting absence figures needs to be studied in more depth. Some studies use percentage absence figures, other mean absence rates and other look at peaks. What works best might be context specific, so what works best in each situation needs to be ascertained. Aldridge et al. (2016) showed how recording of this data could be automated, with an electronic method of submission by schools being used which greatly facilitated data interpretation. Cheng et al. (2012) presented an automatic system for recording such absences. Up to now studies mainly describe only pilots, with most retrospectively showing an association between absenteeism and disease. The next logical step is to show that such data can pre-empt outbreaks and provide forewarning, rather than showing a relationship afterwards. More examination at the effectiveness of this type of data at a local level is needed, such as provided in the study by Besculides et al. (2005) where spatial analysis was used to determine where clusters of absenteeism were occurring.

REFERENCES

Aldridge RW, Hayward AC, Field N, Warren-Gash C, Smith C, Pebody R, Fleming D, McCracken S, Decipher My Data Project and schools. Are school absences correlated with influenza surveillance data in England? Results from Decipher my Data—a research project conducted through scientific engagement with schools. *Plos one.* 2016;**11**(3):e0146964.

Besculides M, Heffernan R, Mostashari F, Weiss D: Evaluation of school absenteeism data for early outbreak detection, New York City. *BMC public health.* 2005;**5**:105-10.

Bollaerts K, Antoine J, Robesyn E, Van Proeyen L, Vomberg J, Feys E, De Decker E, Catry B. Timeliness of syndromic influenza surveillance through work and school absenteeism. *Archives of public health.* 2010;**68**(3):1-6.

Cheng CK, Cowling BJ, Lau EH, Ho LM, Leung GM, Ip DK. Electronic school absenteeism monitoring and influenza surveillance, Hong Kong. *Emerging infectious diseases.* 2012;**18**(5):885.

Crawford GB, McKelvey S, Crooks J, Siska K, Russo K, Chan J. Influenza and school-based influenza-like illness surveillance: a pilot initiative in Maryland. *Public health report.* 2011;**126**:591-6.

Kara EO, Elliot AJ, Bagnall H, Foord DGF, Pnaiser R, Osman H, Smith GE, Olowokure B. Absenteeism in schools during the 2009 influenza A(H1N1) pandemic: a useful tool for early detection of influenza activity in the community? *Epidemiology and infection.* 2011;**140**:1-9.

Kom Mogto CA, De Serres G, Douville Fradet M, Lebel G, Toutant S, Gilca R, Ouakki M, Janjua NZ, Skowronski DM. School absenteeism as an adjunct surveillance indicator: experience during the second wave of the 2009 H1N1 pandemic in Quebec, Canada. *Plos one.* 2012;**7**(3):e34084.

Lenaway DD, Ambler A. Evaluation of a school-based influenza surveillance system. *Public health report.* 1995;**110**: 333-337.

Ma T, Englund H, Bjelkmar P, Wallensten A, Hulth A. Syndromic surveillance of influenza activity in Sweden: an evaluation of three tools. *Epidemiology and infection.* 2015;**143**(11):2390-8.

Mann P, O'Connell E, Zhang G, Llau A, Rico E, Leguen FC. Alert system to detect possible school-based outbreaks of influenza-like illness. *Emerging infectious diseases.* 2011;**17**(2):262-4.

Proctor ME, Blair KA, Davis JP. Surveillance data for waterborne illness detection: an assessment following a massive waterborne outbreak of Cryptosporidium infection. *Epidemiology and infection.* 1998;**120**:43-54.

Sasaki A, Hoen AG, Ozonoff A, Suzuki H, Tanabe N, Seki N, Saito R, Brownstein JS. Evidence-based tool for triggering school closures during influenza outbreaks, Japan. *Emerging infectious diseases.* 2009;**15**(11):1841.

Schmidt WP, Pebody R, Mangtani P. School absence data for influenza surveillance: A pilot study in the United Kingdom. *Eurosurveillance.* 2010;**15**:19467.

Song XX, Zhao Q, Tao T, Zhou CM, Diwan VK, Xu B. Applying the zero-inflated Poisson model with random effects to detect abnormal rises in school absenteeism indicating infectious diseases outbreak. *Epidemiology and infection.* 2018;**146**(12):1565-71.

Suzue T, Hoshikawa Y, Nishihara S, Fujikawa A, Miyatake N, Sakano N, Yoda T, Yoshioka A, Hirao T. The new school absentees reporting system for pandemic influenza A/H1N1 2009 infection in Japan. *Plos one.* 2012;**7**(2):e30639.

Walker MD, Sulyok M. Internet searching on the head louse in the UK since the COVID-19 pandemic. *Pediatric dermatology.* 2023; 40(1):96-99.

Williams NJ, Ghosh TS, Bisgard KM, Vogt RL. Comparison of 3 school-based influenza surveillance indicators: lessons learned from 2009 pandemic influenza a (H1N1)-Denver metropolitan region, Colorado. *Journal of public health management and practise.* 2013;**19**(2):119-25.

Zhao H, Joseph CA, Phin N. Outbreaks of influenza and influenza-like illness in schools in England and Wales, 2005/06. *Eurosurveillance.* 2007;**12**(5):3-4.

13

SMARTPHONES

'Joel, I'm calling you on a cellphone, but a real cellphone, a personal, handheld portable cellphone.'

Marty Cooper, of Motorola making the first public cellphone call to Joel Engel, his AT&T rival. April 1973.

Mobile phones have revolutionized society, providing the possibility of truly personal communication by everyone (Klemens, 2014). Although they were invented in the early 1970's, mobile phones only began being used widely within society from the late 1990's onwards. By the 2010's ownership of mobile phones had become effectively ubiquitous in the Western developed world. 95% of the U.K. population owned one by 2015 (OffCom, 2015).

However, it is arguably in the developing world where the impact of such technology has been greatest because communication using other methods was previously so difficult (Poushter and Stewart, 2016). Mobile phones have allowed easy communication between people living in remote areas where establishing fixed lines would be completely uneconomic (Etzo and Collender, 2010). From an epidemiological viewpoint this is important because it is these areas which continue to be challenged by the most pernicious of infectious diseases such as malaria.

Another leap forwards came with the development of smartphones which allowed access to the internet. Smartphone ownership in the U.K. had risen to over 66% by 2014 from only 39% in 2012 (OffCom, 2015). On average mobile phone users were spending over two hours per day accessing the internet through their phone in 2014. The figure is undoubtedly even higher now. Although conventional mobile phones simply facilitated communication, the internet connectivity that smartphones allowed has opened up many new exiting possibilities. For example, the integration of features such as digital cameras along with internet access has opened up the possibility of photographic based disease testing in the field with diagnosis being confirmed remotely through accessing specially conceived apps.

How have mobile phones and smartphones aided epidemiology?
Healthcare professionals were quick to adopt mobile phones (Choi et al. 2012). Among the many tasks which mobile phones have helped in the healthcare arena include:

- **Management of patient records:** Phones with internet access open up the possibility of clinicians updating patient records remotely, and pretty much as soon as they see a patient. This is likely to lead to increased accuracy, with instant updating of records meaning mistakes are less likely to occur as can be the case if records are paper based and updated later. Also, crucially from a disease surveillance point of view, epidemiologists can now access data much easier and quicker meaning they obtain information about potential disease outbreaks promptly (Reviewed: Ventola et al. 2014).

- **Better diagnosis:** Traditionally diagnosis relied on a clinicians knowledge and experience. The availability of phones with internet access meant healthcare professionals can obtain information instantly from appropriate websites, even while at the patient bedside. There was no need to refer to possibly outdated books or journals. Instead an up-to-date website or journal article could be consulted. Another development were various apps specially conceived to aid diagnosis. Better diagnosis helps those studying disease as it means a quicker, more accurate picture of the disease situation is available, allowing the ability to potentially spot outbreaks quicker.

- **Improved communication, improved connectivity:** Mobile devices have greatly facilitated communication, meaning clinicians can phone, email or text colleagues about problems, experiences, ideas or simply to ask for help. Prue et al. (2013), for example, showed how mobile phones improved reporting of malaria in rural Bangladesh, increasing reports of suspected illness, and the requesting of testing and treatments. News about potential outbreaks can spread quicker meaning those on the ground are aware of potential problems and can thus be on the look out for them. Previously, when an outbreak occurred, even medical professionals in close proximity could remain totally unaware of it.

- **Patient participation:** It is not only clinicians who have access to more information, but patients and potential patients too. As described elsewhere in this book, people are willing to use personal health 'apps' to improve their own well-being. This means the general population has increased knowledge of health care issues, potential problems, and what to look out for. There are effectively now more eyes on the ground than before. For example, during the initial phases of COVID-19 pandemic, knowledge about potential symptoms spread globally very quickly. Epidemiology has become increasingly democratized.

Examples of where mobile phones aid epidemiology
Mobile phones have aided disease surveillance simply by speeding up and improving communication. This means that notification of potential disease cases can be done almost instantaneously. But are there any specific examples where mobile phones have been used directly to help disease surveillance?

One example is that provided by Robertson (2010). Field veterinarians in Sri Lanka are required to fill out health surveys related to the animals they encounter and the diseases they harbour. In this study the field veterinarians trialled using mobile phones to send filled out survey forms, with them

135

being relayed to a central administrator. Although this study concentrated on diseases in chickens, cattle, and buffalo, it was one of the first which showed the potential of mobile phones for the relaying of disease surveillance data in remote and poor areas of the world where other methods of communication would be slow or unreliable.

SMS: TEXTING AND DISEASE

A great feature of the new mobile phones was the ability to send text messages; Short Message Service- SMS's. This allowed the relaying of short textual pieces of information between mobile phone users. In a review article Zurovac et al. (2012) identified the great potential SMS texting offered for disease surveillance, particularly in Africa and the management of malaria. The authors noted that a key benefit was cost; with the sending of texts being minimal. They also noted that this technology was available to anyone with a mobile phone, unlike more advanced features which required expensive handsets and devices with internet connectivity.

Randriosolo et al. (2010) reported on a sentinel system for the reporting of chikungunya in Madagascar using SMS's. Sentinel General Practitioners provided detailed reports on patients through conventional form filling. However, the system was supplemented with the use of SMS. Medics sent daily texts detailing the number of cases of fever they had seen, and the number of confirmed cases of malaria and other similar febrile illnesses. Trialling of the system began in March 2007, and during 2008 five outbreaks across 13 health districts were identified and reported using the SMS system. This showed the ability of SMS to aid the prompt reporting of outbreaks.

Attempts have been made to overcome the limited amount of information that can be sent by texts by developing codes that enable more detailed information to be sent in a shortened format. A method for sending detailed information using such shortened coded formats was demonstrated by Asiimwe et al. (2011). A SMS based surveillance system for malaria was established in the Gulul and Kabala districts of Uganda. A method was devised to standardize data, which was then sent in a SMS to a central 'RapidSMS' processing system. This automatically collated data and processed the texts meaning useful feedback was obtained.

Another example of how texting could help malaria surveillance was provided by Githinji et al (2014). Malaria was assessed across 87 Kenyan healthcare facilities, with professionals required to text information related to cases to a central administrator using SMS. This study showed that although response rates were high, the accuracy of data sent was not, which is probably not surprising given the low level of content that can be included in such texts. This early study suggested that texts alone were not sufficient for such surveillance, but could be a useful addition.

Although the potential of SMS texting was investigated, and seemed initially promising, its use for disease surveillance became somewhat redundant with the increasing ease of obtaining internet connectivity. It became easier to email information, which allowed more detail to be sent, or latterly submit data through the use of specially conceived 'apps'.

THE RISE OF THE 'APPS'

The use of 'apps' has become increasingly prevalent. An 'app', short for application, is simply a piece of software that helps perform some specific task. They are easily installed on a desktop computer, a smartphone, or tablet, or can be accessed directly through the web. Mobile apps designed for smartphones are typically simpler and easier to use than the desktop versions, meaning they are easier to use on-the-go without a keyboard.

A variety of apps providing a range of online health services intended for use by the general public have been developed. Such apps have gained great popularity in recent years. Increasingly they are able to be used in conjunction with 'wearables', such as smartwatches, which automatically monitor body status and can upload data to the app automatically. This allows personalized and specific health advice to be provided. The classic example would be the weight loss app, which provides advice for suggested diets and exercise routines. 'MyHealthyday', for example, was founded in 2001 by Andrew Sherman. This online site stores your health information in one place and allows users to monitor health parameters through a smartwatch. Such personal apps have found much use in the management of chronic diseases.

Such personal apps designed for the general public have opened up a new research avenue for epidemiologists wanting to obtain data upon specific interest groups. However, one problem potentially limiting such research is that users of such technology tend to be aggregated among certain socio-demographic groups such as the young and highly educated (Carroll et al. 2017). However, as the technology becomes more widespread this is likely to change. Studies examining the effectiveness of such apps in improving personal health are mixed (Zhao et al. 2016).

There are other potential problems with such systems. These apps are typically developed by private companies with profit motives. The apps rely on individuals providing potentially sensitive personal information about themselves, which is then processed for use by a larger community. This raises issues relating to anonymity and data privacy. Do users really know what data is being used for, and who might have access to it?

Apps for disease surveillance

Are there any apps specifically conceived for disease surveillance and epidemic monitoring? A review by Mohanty et al. (2019) collated information on various health apps and assessed their use and potential for this. Over 100 health related apps were identified and examined, with 26 being found to be centred on the surveillance of disease. Most were intended for the general public, rather than medical professionals. Key features they often included were interactive maps, the ability to track infections, and the ability to receive alerts. The most popular was found to be HealthMap, described in a previous chapter. Most apps concentrated on a single disease or condition. Overall the authors concluded that apps offer great potential for disease surveillance if developed further.

The source of information behind these apps varied. HealthMap, for example, uses a range of input sources including PROMed mail and Google News. Another popular app, FluView, uses information from the CDC Influenza Surveillance Network. Many disease apps do not use user provided data or information, instead acting more as information hubs, collating information from elsewhere then providing maps and updates to users as to trends or potential outbreaks. Examples include FluMapTracker and ViralMap. FluTrack monitors tweets for mention of influenza.

Of great potential interest are those which collect data from user participants, often called 'crowdsourcing' or 'participatory' apps, with member information being processed and integrated into disease tracking. Of such apps based predominately on user inputted data is Sickweather, which is the largest and most well known. A preponderance of such apps examine influenza. The overwhelming geographical emphasis of these apps is the western developed world. However, of note are apps for conditions of relevance in the developing world such as Zika virus and dengue fever.

Example participatory apps of use for disease surveillance which use crowdsourced data, adapted from Mohanty et al. (2019)

'app'	Reference	State.
Flu near you	Smolinksi et al. (2015)	U.S.
Influenzanet	Koppeschaar et al (2017)	Europe wide
Flureport	Fujibahyashi et al (2018)	Japan
Flutracking	Dalton et al. (2017)	Australia

Selected examples of participatory apps:

Apps for the 2014 World Cup and 2016 Olympic Games: An interesting example of apps specifically conceived for disease surveillance is provided by those developed for the 2014 FIFA World Cup and the 2016 Olympic Games

'HealthyCup' was a participatory disease surveillance app implemented during the FIFA Football World Cup held in Brazil in 2014 (Neto et al. 2017). This app involved public collaboration to monitor three syndromes; respiratory, diarrhoeal, and rash. These could be an indication of six important diseases that epidemiologists wanted to monitor during the event; influenza, measles, rubella, cholera, acute diarrhoea, and dengue fever. Users who downloaded the app reported if they were ill or well, and if they were not well they then answered a serious of questions related to their symptoms. There were over 7,000 users of the app. 4,700 who were active. Although this was small in scale, it showed the promise of such app usage in monitoring potential disease outbreaks during such high profile events with a large number of spectators who had travelled across the globe to reach it.

Following on from this, in 2016, the Guardiões da Saúde (Guardians of Health) app, was developed to study disease outbreaks during the 2016 Rio Olympic Games (Neto et al. 2020). Participants were questioned as to their location and about a strategically chosen list of symptoms that could indicate diarrhoeal, respiratory, and rash based illnesses. Use of daily prompts and games prompted users to provide information on a daily basis. The ultimate aim was to track potential outbreaks of the infectious conditions chikungunya, Zika virus and dengue fever. Although gaining more users than HealthyCup, this study highlighted that such apps face problems of user recruitment and engagement. From 59,312 downloads, only 7,848 became users, with only 5,980 of these using it more than once. The use of quizzes was not enough to engage people.

Sickweather: Maybe the most well known citizen science participatory app is Sickweather (Sickweather, 2023). Founded in 2011 by Graham Dodge, Michael Belt and James Sajor. Sickweather is specifically designed as an illness tracking app. It processes reports of illness submitted either by registered members, but also includes mention of important disease related keywords by users of social media sites such as Facebook or Twitter. If you are signed up, it messages you when you enter a location where specific disease might occur, or when an outbreak happens near to where you are. Are you entering a 'flu' hotspot? It is cited as processing six million reports of illness each month. The British Lung Foundation has recommended its use for those with conditions such as asthma and bronchitis, as it advised on weather conditions which might potentially exacerbate symptoms. An additional feature of interest to the epidemiologist is that Sickweather uses machine learning methods, with the data it obtains being used to make forecasts about the future number of potential disease cases.

Appdemia: A similar participatory app to Sickweather is Appdemia, where users can record symptoms and the conditions they have, and these are used to inform the wider community.

Outbreaks near me: This participatory app was developed from the earlier 'Flu Near Me' app by researchers at Boston Children's Hospital and Harvard University. Participants are asked to provide details of symptoms they have experienced, which are then mapped, thus showing potential influenza hotspots. During the COVID-19 pandemic a version entitled 'COVID Near You' was developed. 'Outbreaks Near Me' now provides mapping for both influenza and COVID-19, as can be seen on the provided illustration.

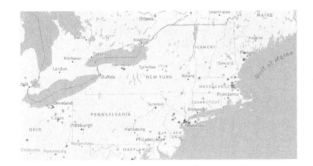 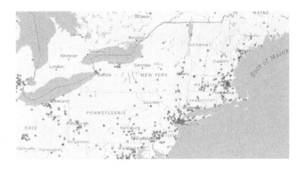

Maps from Outbreaks Near Me, obtained from August 2022 showing (left) self reported influenza symptoms, (right) self reported COVID-19 symptoms, over a three week period for New York and Pennsylvania States.

SORMAS and Ebola surveillance: Ebola is a condition where rapid identification and control of cases is the best way of stopping rapid transmission and reducing the size of the ultimate outbreak. Can apps help to nip outbreaks in the bud? A great number have been developed with Ebola in mind (Tom-Aba, et al. 2018). One example is SORMAS (Surveillance and Outbreak Response

Management System), which was developed in conjunction with the German Helmholz centre. This allows identification and management of Ebola cases (Fähnrich et al. 2015).

FeverCoach: The Korean FeverCoach app is a good example how patient care can be combined with the collection of data for epidemiological purposes. Parents with children under five who appear to be suffering from influenza can register for the app, and on providing details of their child receive treatment and care advice. Researchers used submitted data to model the likely number of influenza cases, finding that predictions made with FeverCoach data mirrored official data from the Korean Center for Disease Control. Additionally, there was evidence that FeverCoach data predicted an epidemic 10 days earlier than official data (Kim et al. 2019).

MOSapp and DISapp: Dengue is a huge problem in India, this country having the largest number of cases worldwide. The development of an early warning and adaptive response system called EWARS aimed to spot potential hotspots (Babu et al. 2019). This project is interesting in that it uses a combination of data both from medical professionals and from the general public as well. An app for professionals, MOSapp, allows uploading of environmental factors potentially influencing dengue occurrence. The public based app, DISapp, allows the public to do the same. The public app also plays an educational role, providing information of the risk of dengue at specific locations and preventative measures that can be taken. This dual approach means much greater data can be collected than simply using either medical professional or public alone.

Argus: El Khatib et al. (2018) reported on on the effectiveness of an app called Argus, conceived for one area of the Central African Republic, Mambéré Kadéi. It was found that its use increased reporting on conditions and this could aid disease surveillance. The Argus app has three functions; alerting of potential outbreaks, reporting of weekly and monthly cases, and a final function allowing archiving of cases for future retrieval.

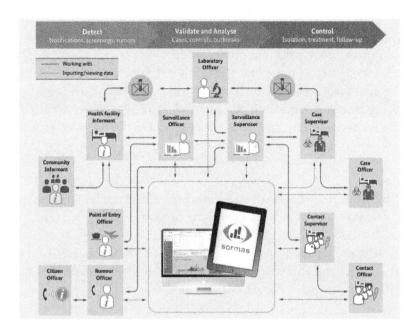

SORMAS: Image showing the range of people inputting and utilising the SORMAS Ebola app. Image taken from 'A software for disease surveillance and outbreak response' by the German Health Consortium, 2020. https://health.bmz.de/wp-content/uploads/studies/GHPC_SORMAS_full_version_final.pdf

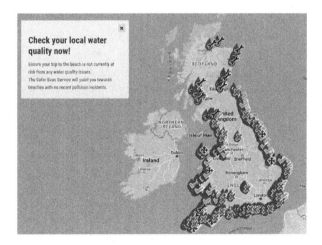

The charity 'Surfers against Sewage' provide an app allowing users to monitor U.K. water quality. An interactive map using real-time CSOs (combined sewage overflows) and PRFs (pollution risk forecasts) shows water quality at 400 locations around U.K. rivers and coast-lines. Such resources could be used in conjunction with disease surveillance data to study the relationship between environmental factors and outbreaks of water borne disease. Available at: www.sas.org.uk/map/

SMILE CAMERA!

Another feature of modern smartphones is the ability to take photos with a built in camera. The quality of these is excellent and now often exceeds that possible using older traditional cameras. Another bonus, is that such images can be easily sent using the very same phone that has taken them. This phone-as-a-camera opens up the possibility of improving disease diagnosis. A number of conditions can be diagnosed on the basis of images. This has a knock on consequence for epidemiology.

Vector identification

One example of the ability of cameras to take and send high quality images comes from entomology and the study of vector-borne diseases. In one project, a citizen science 'e-entomology' project in southern Australia used such images (Sousa et al. 2020). Pictures of mosquitoes caught at 126 fixed trapping points were emailed to entomologists at a central location for identification. This allowed changes in the seasonal abundance of mosquitoes to be ascertained, which could be importance in anticipating problems with vector borne conditions.

Phone as microscope

The camera present in mobile phones can be used as an ersatz microscope, allowing samples to be studied and diagnosis be made on the spot. In remote areas of the developing world, where diagnostic equipment is costly or difficult to obtain, this is an important potential use. A magnifying lens needs to be attached to the camera for it to be used as a microscope, allowing images to be enlarged enough for analysis. This has been investigated in a number of studies.

Often cited, is Bogoch et al. (2014) where researchers attached a small lens to the camera of an Apple mobile phone for the the identification of *Schistosoma mansoni* parasites in the stool samples of school aged children. Ephraim et al. (2016) showed how a lens added to the phone could aid identification of Schistosome eggs in child urine. Coulibaly et al. (2016) added a small microscope to a phone to help identification of plasmodium parasites in samples. These studies required the manual assessment of samples, but it is also possible to develop automatic systems to analyse images. Slusaweric et al. (2016) used image recognition software to automatically count numbers of parasitic eggs in stool samples.

Study	Details
D'Ambrosio et al. (2015)	Developed a mobile phone–based video microscope to measure the *Loa loa* microfilariae in blood samples, to decide who received Ivermectin drug treatment.
Pirnstill and Coté (2015)	Introduced a polarized microscope to help in the diagnosis of malaria.
Sowerby et al. (2016)	A Nokia Lumia 1020 with an additional objective lens was used to examine *Ascaris lumbricoides* eggs.
Rosado et al. (2016)	Blood smears were examined by smartphone cameras for presence of *Plasmodium falciparum* trophozoites.

SMART DIAGNOSTICS

Another way in which mobile phones can be used for on-the-spot diagnosis is where they are used in conjunction with other testing devices to detect a pathogen. A variety of such testing kits exist. They are known properly as Rapid Diagnostic Tests, but often more informally known as 'lab on a chip' devices. Perhaps the most commonly encountered example of Rapid Diagnostic Tests most people know about are the rapid COVID-19 home testing kits, or home pregnancy kits, which both allow quick and easy diagnosis.

Mobile phones can be used with such testing kit, with for example a smartphone flash providing the light source, and the camera being used as a detector or recording device.

Diagnosing Zika

Ganguli et al (2017) used Smartphone technology to aid the diagnosis of Zika virus. This vector borne condition is transmitted mainly by female *Aedes aegypti* mosquitoes. It occurs across tropical areas of the globe, notably across south America, sub-Saharan Africa and the Indian subcontinent. A problem is that diagnosis based on symptoms is ineffective, as many of the symptoms mirror those of other conditions. Additionally, Zika mainly occurs in rural areas and among the poor where diagnosis is limited. What is needed is diagnosis on the spot, in the field. Effectively spotting cases is especially important because it means outbreaks can be nipped in the bud before cases multiply. Diagnosis of a single patient can potentially prevent many more becoming infected.

Researchers tasked with improving diagnosis developed a pre-printed chip, a 'lab-on-a-chip' to use their own wording. This allowed the analysis of a blood sample, with amplification of any viral RNA occurring if it was present. A smartphone could then be used to photograph the amplification reaction, which could then be analysed and a diagnosis made.

Example studies of Smartphones being used in conjunction with lab-on-a-chips

Study	Details
Guo et al. (2021)	Demonstrated a system for species specific testing of malaria. Used paper-based microfluidic lateral flow diagnostic test . The testing device was powered and controlled via mobile phone. Results analysed via the phone and a cloud based 'app' for diagnosis using machine learning Algorithms and a Blockchain for security. Effectiveness demonstrated in a trial in Uganda..
Stemple et al. (2016)	Utilised the flash as a light source and the phone camera as the detector, for a lab-on-a-chip for the detection of malaria antigents in blood samples.
Scherr et al. (2014)	Used a mobile phone camera to take images of Rapid Diagnostic Tests for malaria. Once uploaded to a database called REDCap, automated image processing program assessed them.

MEASURING MOBILITY

Human mobility and disease transmission are intrinsically linked. It is intuitive that the more people move around, the more likely the infectious conditions they harbour will be transmitted to new people. This has long been known; attempts at restricting movement to stop the spread of disease date back centuries. The name 'quarantine' originates with attempts to stop spread of plague by limiting movement.

However, actually demonstrating a link between mobility and disease empirically is much more challenging. It is difficult to track people's movements. Logistically monitoring personal movements exactly is difficult to do in terms of time and resources.

Mobile phones provide a possibility to do this. A simple method is to monitor call location. Mobile phone companies record calls made by individual users. Calls can be monitored as to which local areas they occur within, centred on central mobile phone towers or cases. This allows the possibility of recording should a user move from one area to another. However, this relies on the owner of the phone actually making telephone calls when they move to a new location. Increasingly it is becoming possible to actually track movement even if this is not the case; Bluetooth and global positioning allows any movement to be detected and recorded.

A clutch of studies examining mobility using mobile phone records and disease appeared in the 2010's. Already a classic is that by Wesolowski et al. (2012) which examined patterns of human movement and malaria spread using mobile phone data from Kenya. Those infected with malaria can carry the disease to new areas. This study used the data from 15 million Kenyan cell phone users, with users being assigned a primary settlement. The amount of movement from primary settlements was measured and using malaria prevalence maps the chances of malaria being carried to other areas was modelled and then predicted

Studies using mobile phone records to study mobility and disease

Study	Details
Bengtsson et al. (2015)	Used mobile phone records to assess levels of mobility and study its relationship with outbreaks of cholera using data from the Haittian Cholera outbreak of 2010.
Isdory et al. (2015)	Integrated mobility data obtained from mobile phone records into SIR models for HIV in different regions of Kenya.
Wesolowski et al. (2015)	Modelled the climatic and mobility dynamics of dengue fever in Pakistan using mobile records and found they mirrored what happened in a 2013 outbreak.
Zhu et al. (2019)	Modelled dengue fever using mobility and temperature data, and found that mobility data spatial transmission across cities.

144

REFERENCES

Asiimwe C, Gelvin D, Lee E, Amor YB, Quinto E, Katureebe C, Sundaram L, Bell D, Berg M. Use of an innovative, affordable, and open-source short message service–based tool to monitor malaria in remote areas of Uganda. *The American journal of tropical medicine and hygiene.* 2011;**85**(1):26.

Babu AN, Niehaus E, Shah S, Unnithan C, Ramkumar PS, Shah J, Binoy VV, Soman B, Arunan MC, Jose CP. Smartphone geospatial apps for dengue control, prevention, prediction, and education: MOSapp, DISapp, and the mosquito perception index (MPI). *Environmental monitoring and assessment.* 2019;**191**(2):1-7.

Bengtsson L, Gaudart J, Lu X, Moore S, Wetter E, Sallah K, Rebaudet S, Piarroux R. Using mobile phone data to predict the spatial spread of cholera. *Scientific reports.* 2015;**5**(1):1-5.

Bogoch II, Coulibaly JT, Andrews JR, Speich B, Keiser J, Stothard JR, N'Goran EK, Utzinger J. Evaluation of portable microscopic devices for the diagnosis of *Schistosoma* and soil-transmitted helminth infection. *Parasitology.* 2014;**141**:1811-1818.

Carroll JK, Moorhead A, Bond R, LeBlanc WG, Petrella RJ, Fiscella K. Who uses mobile phone health apps and does use matter? A secondary data analytics approach. *Journal of medical internet research.* 2017;**19**;19(4):e5604.

Choi JS, Yi B, Park JH, Choi K, Jung J, Park SW, Rhee P. The uses of the smartphone for doctors: An empirical study from Samsung medical center. *Healthcare information research.* 2011;**17**(2):131–138.

Coulibaly JT, Ouattara M, Keiser J, Bonfoh B, N'Goran EK, Andrews JR, Bogoch II. Evaluation of malaria diagnoses using a handheld light microscope in a community-based setting in rural Cote d'Ivoire. *American journal of tropical medicine and hygiene.* 2016; **95**:831-834.

Dalton C, Carlson S, Butler M, Cassano D, Clarke S, Fejsa J, Durrheim D. Insights from flutracking: thirteen tips to growing a web-based participatory surveillance system. *JMIR public health and surveillance.* 2017;**3**(3):e7333.

D'Ambrosio MV, Bakalar M, Bennuru S, Reber C, Skandarajah A, Nilsson L, Switz N, Kamgno J, Pion S, Boussinesq M, Nutman TB. Point-of-care quantification of blood-borne filarial parasites with a mobile phone microscope. *Science translational medicine.* 2015;**7**(286):286re4-.

El-Khatib Z, Shah M, Zallappa SN, Nabeth P, Guerra J, Manengu CT, Yao M, Philibert A, Massina L, Staiger CP, Mbailao R. SMS-based smartphone application for disease surveillance has doubled completeness and timeliness in a limited-resource setting–evaluation of a 15-week pilot program in Central African Republic (CAR). *Conflict and health.* 2018;**12**(1):1-1.

Ephraim RKD, Duah E, Cybulski JS, Prakash M, D'Ambrosio MV, Fletcher DA, Keiser J, Andrews JR, Bogoch II. Diagnosis of *Schistosoma haematobium* infection with a mobile phone-mounted Foldscope and a reversed-lens CellScope in Ghana. *American journal of tropical medicine and hygiene.* **2016;**92:1253-1256.

Etzo S, Collender G. The mobile phone 'revolution' in Africa: rhetoric or reality?. *African affairs.* 2010;**109**(437):659-68.

Fähnrich C, Denecke K, Adeoye O O, Benzler J, Claus H, Kirchner G, Mall S, Richter R, Schapranow M P, Schwarz NG, Tom-Aba D, Uflacker M, Poggensee G, Krause G. Surveillance and Outbreak Response Management System (SORMAS) to support the control of the Ebola virus disease outbreak in West Africa. *Eurosurveillance.* 2015;**20**(12):pii=21071.

Fujibayashi K, Takahashi H, Tanei M, Uehara Y, Yokokawa H, Naito T. A new influenza-tracking smartphone app (flu-report) based on a self-administered questionnaire: cross-sectional study. *JMIR mhealth and uhealth.* 2018;**6**(6):e136.

Githinji S, Kigen S, Memusi D, Nyandigisi A, Wamari A, Muturi A, Jagoe G, Ziegler R, Snow RW, Zurovac D. Using mobile phone text messaging for malaria surveillance in rural Kenya. *Malaria journal.* 2014;**13**(1):1-9.

Guo X, Khalid MA, Domingos I, Michala AL, Adriko M, Rowel C, Ajambo D, Garrett A, Kar S, Yan X, Reboud J. Smartphone-based DNA diagnostics for malaria detection using deep learning for local decision support and blockchain technology for security. *Nature electronics.* 2021;**4**(8):615-24.

Isdory A, Mureithi EW, Sumpter DJ. The impact of human mobility on HIV transmission in Kenya. *Plos one.* 2015;**10**(11):e0142805.

Klemens G. The cellphone: The history and technology of the gadget that changed the world. McFarland; 2014.

Kim M, Yune S, Chang S, Jung Y, Sa S, Han H. The fever coach mobile app for participatory influenza surveillance in children: usability study. *JMIR mHealth uHealth.* 2019;**7**(10):e14276

Koppeschaar CE, Colizza V, Guerrisi C, Turbelin C, Duggan J, Edmunds WJ, Kjelsø C, Mexia R, Moreno Y, Meloni S, Paolotti D. Influenzanet: citizens among 10 countries collaborating to monitor influenza in Europe. *JMIR public health and surveillance.* 2017;**3**(3):e7429.

Mohanty B, Chughtai A, Rabhi F. Use of Mobile Apps for epidemic surveillance and response–availability and gaps. *Global biosecurity.* 2019;**1**(1).

Neto OL, Cruz O, Albuquerque J, de Sousa MN, Smolinski M, Cesse EÂ, Libel M, de Souza WV. Participatory surveillance based on crowdsourcing during the Rio 2016 Olympic Games using the guardians of health platform: descriptive study. *JMIR public health and surveillance.* 2020;**6**(2):e16119.

Neto OL, Dimech GS, Libel M, de Souza WV, Cesse E, Smolinski M, Oliveira W, Albuquerque J. Saúde na copa: the world's first application of participatory surveillance for a mass gathering at FIFA World Cup 2014, Brazil. *JMIR public health and surveillance.* 2017;**3**(2):e7313.

OffCom. The Communications Market Report 2015. Available at: www.ofcom.org.uk/research-and-data/multi-sector-research/cmr/cmr15

Pirnstill CW, Coté GL. Malaria diagnosis using a mobile phone polarized microscope. *Scientific reports.* 2015;**5**(1):1-3.

Poushter J, Stewart R. Smartphone ownership and internet usage continues to climb in emerging economies - but advanced economies still have higher rates of technology use. Pew Research Center. 2016. Available at: http://www.pewglobal.org/2016/02/22/smartphone-ownership-and-internet-usage-continues-to-climb-in-emerging-economies/

Prue CS, Shannon KL, Khyang J, Edwards LJ, Ahmed S, Ram M, Shields T, Hossain MS, Glass GE, Nyunt MM, Sack DA. Mobile phones improve case detection and management of malaria in rural Bangladesh. *Malaria journal.* 2013;**12**(1):1-7.

Randrianasolo L, Raoelina Y, Ratsitorahina M, Ravolomanana L, Andriamandimby S, Heraud JM, Rakotomanana F, Ramanjato R, Randrianarivo-Solofoniaina AE, Richard V. Sentinel surveillance system for early outbreak detection in Madagascar. *BMC public health.* 2010;**10**:31.

Robertson C, Sawford K, Daniel SL, Nelson TA, Stephen C. Mobile phone–based infectious disease surveillance system, Sri Lanka. *Emerging infectious diseases.* 2010;**16**(10):1524.

Rosado L, da Costa JMC, Elias D, Cardoso JS. Automated detection of malaria parasites on thick blood smears via mobile devices. *Procedia computer science.* 2016;**90**;138-144.

Scherr TF, Gupta S, Wright DW, Haselton FR. Mobile phone imaging and cloud-based analysis for standardized malaria detection and reporting. *Scientific reports.* 2016;**6**(1):1-9.

Sickweather. How Sickweather Works. 2022. Available at: http://www.sickweather.com/how/
Slusarewicz P, Pagano S, Mills C, Popa G, Chow KM, Mendenhall M, Rodgers DW, Nielsen MK. Automated parasite faecal egg counting using fluorescence labelling, smartphone image capture and computational image analysis. *International journal of parasitology.* 2016:**46**;485-493.

Smolinski MS, Crawley AW, Baltrusaitis K, Chunara R, Olsen JM, Wójcik O, Santillana M, Nguyen A, Brownstein JS. Flu near you: crowdsourced symptom reporting spanning 2 influenza seasons. *American journal of public health.* 2015;**105**(10):2124-30.

Sowerby SJ, Crump JA, Johnstone MC, Krause KL, Hill PC. Smartphone microscopy of parasite eggs accumulated into a single field of view. *The American journal of tropical medicine and hygiene.* 2016;**94**(1):227.

Sousa LB, Fricker SR, Doherty SS, Webb CE, Baldock KL, Williams CR. Citizen science and smartphone e-entomology enables low-cost upscaling of mosquito surveillance. *Science of the total environment.* 2020;**704**:135349.

Stemple CC, Angus SV, Park TS, Yoon JY. Smartphone-based optofluidic lab-on-a-chip for detecting pathogens from blood. *Journal of laboratory automation.* 2014;**19**(1):35-41.

Tom-Aba D, Nguku PM, Arinze CC, Krause G. Assessing the Concepts and Designs of 58 Mobile Apps for the Management of the 2014-2015 West Africa Ebola Outbreak: Systematic Review. *JMIR public health surveillance.* 2018;**4**(4):e68.

Ventola CL. Mobile devices and apps for health care professionals: uses and benefits. *Pharmacy and therapeutics.* 2014;**39**(5):356.

Wesolowski A, Qureshi T, Boni MF, Sundsøy PR, Johansson MA, Rasheed SB, Engø-Monsen K, Buckee CO. Impact of human mobility on the emergence of dengue epidemics in Pakistan. *Proceedings of the national academy of sciences.* 2015;**112**(38):11887-92.

Wesolowski A, Eagle N, Tatem AJ, Smith DL, Noor AM, Snow RW, Buckee CO. Quantifying the impact of human mobility on malaria. *Science.* 2012;**338**(6104):267-70.

Zhao J, Freeman B, Li M. Can mobile phone apps influence people's health behavior change? An evidence review. *Journal of medical internet research.* 2016;**18**(11):e5692.

Zhu G, Liu T, Xiao J, Zhang B, Song T, Zhang Y, Lin L, Peng Z, Deng A, Ma W, Hao Y. Effects of human mobility, temperature and mosquito control on the spatiotemporal transmission of dengue. *Science of the total environment.* 2019;**651**:969-78.

Zurovac D, Talisuna AO, Snow RW. Mobile phone text messaging: tool for malaria control in Africa. *Plos medicine.* 2012;**9**(2):e1001176.

14

TWITTER

On Twitter, we get excited if someone follows us.
In real life, we get really scared and run away .

Anonymous.

One message, 140 characters. The underlying idea of Twitter is to convey an idea, a message, or news, as shortly and quickly as possible. This tallies well with the ethos of the modern age, which values the instantaneous and induces ever shortening attention spans. Friends Jack Dorsey, Noah Glass, Biz Stone, and Evan Williams developed Twitter in March 2006. It was launched later that same year. The underlying idea behind Twitter had been used in a version named 'Odio' from 2004.

Twitter is an example of a 'microblog'. These are sites which allow users to post messages, follow the messages posted by others they are interested in, and effectively be part of online communities. They offer users the opportunity to describe what they are doing, how they are feeling and their general attitude to life. In some respects microblogs can be considered as a public form of diary, allowing people to connect with people worldwide in a way that has never been possible before. Twitter is only one example of such a microblog. Others which exist include Facebook, Instagram, and Pinterest. These allow the posting of pictures as well as text. Collectively these are often referred to as 'social media'.

These social media platforms could offer epidemiologists an ideal additional resource to learn about disease. After all, if users of such platforms are ready to describe how they feel about a politician or pop star, or post a picture of their dinner, then they are also likely to post if they feel unwell and maybe even describe what symptoms they have.

You are what you Tweet
Interest in the use of social media platforms such as Twitter for disease surveillance purposes began in the early 2010's, only a few years after these sites came into existence. The H1N1 influenza pandemic, colloquially known simply as 'swine flu', provided epidemiologists with arguably the first chance to examine whether patterns in messaging with these new technologies reflected disease occurrence in real life.

Maybe the first to examine the relationship between Twitter and disease were researchers Chew and Eysenbach (2010). They analysed two million Tweets containing reference to either 'swine flu' or 'H1N1' and successfully showed that there were Twitter peaks that could be traced to important news media stories. They were also able to show that there was an association between Twitter message numbers and incidence data. They realized the potential of their work in that it could allow effective and easy early tracking of trends in infectious disease outbreaks.

Inevitably, early research using social media platforms concentrated on influenza. A clutch of studies appeared between 2010 and 2013 looking at Tweets about this condition. Notable is the work of Culotta et al. (2010), where over 500,000 Tweets were examined over a ten week period of 2010. They examined mention of both a selection of hand chosen keywords related to influenza ('flu', 'cough', 'sore throat', 'headache'), plus other keywords related to these symptoms. They then fitted data on the usage of these words into regression models and compared the results to official statistics about influenza-like-illness from the U.S. Center for Disease Control. They found that Twitter messages were a promising tool with which to forecast those elusive Winter influenza peaks.

However, it was arguably the seminal article by Paul and Dredze (2011) that gained most attention and raised awareness about the possibilities of using Twitter for infectious disease research. In 'You are What You Tweet' they encouraged more and better use of Twitter for health research purposes. They recognized that Tweets could be used for far more than simply calculating the correlation between disease incidence and Tweet numbers. They realized that despite their brevity, Tweets contained a variety of information of importance to those interested in studying disease. For example, they provide location information, allowing monitoring of where Tweets related to illness were coming from. They might also include details of the treatments being used and which symptoms were experienced by Tweeters.

The language challenge
The principle problem faced by those wishing to use Tweets for research purposes is the sheer volume of messages and the weight of text which requires processing. An estimated 500 million Tweets are sent each day (Post, 2022). Despite their brevity, the number of messages means any researcher trying to study them one-by one would be overwhelmed. Another problem is semantics; word meaning. Those posting Tweets might use a variety of terms to suggest a single meaning; they might use words in a ironic way, or choose words with double meanings. These complexities of language mean that the perceived content of Tweets might be different from their actual meaning. Additionally Tweeters might use a variety of synonyms, describe symptoms others are experiencing and not themselves, or use unclear language.

Aramake et al. (2011) provided some examples of these problems relating to influenza; such as a question posed by one Tweeter:

'Headache? You might have flu'.

This Tweet is referring to illness in another person, not the Tweeter themselves. Obviously, if classifying simply on use of the word 'flu' would mean this was incorrectly classed as a case. The next example shows that messages might contain confusing terms, and is an example of a Tweeted news story:

'The World Health Organization reports the avian influenza, or bird flu, epidemic has spread to nine Asian countries in the past few weeks'

It mentions 'avian influenza', but has nothing to do with human influenza at all. As another example, just think of the phrase:

'I am sick of this'

The Tweet contains the word 'sick', but the Tweeter is not actually ill at all, merely expressing they are fed up with something.

Obviously what is required is some method to filter Tweets and extract those of interest to the researcher. Aramake et al. (2011) developed a vocabulary of phrases, which were indicative that the writer potentially had influenza. They then used a machine learning technique known as Support Vector Machines (SVM) to classify Tweets into those where the writers probably had influenza, and the rest where they probably did not. Machine learning is ideal for such repetitive tasks, simply because of the sheer volume of messages which need classifying.

The authors examined 300 million Tweets, running from November 2008 to June 2010. A problem they encountered was the H1N1 'swine flu' pandemic, which caused what they termed 'news excessive periods'. Large numbers of Tweets not related to actual cases of human influenza were sent. This problem had previously been encountered by Chew and Eysenach (2010). During these periods there was a poor correlation between Tweet numbers and official influenza statistics, whether they examined the method of classifying Tweets they had developed, or simply used the raw frequency of Tweets. However, when they examined the relationship during non-news excessive periods Tweets generally correlated well with the influenza data. The SVM method of classifying Tweets proved to be better than using raw numbers.

Methods for processing language

Much research has been conducted into how statistical computing and machine learning can be used for the processing of text and language. The ability to spot trends and patterns in written language is of use across a wide range of disciplines, including marketing, counter terrorism, social science research, or as is the case here, the study of disease.

Two terms concerned with the analysis of the written language are text mining and natural language processing. Text mining is the name given to the task of managing and extracting information from large amounts of text data. Text mining includes the categorization of texts, ascertaining the text context, summarizing texts, and performing sentiment analysis. This process can be automated, with analysis of news related articles occurring as they are published.

More advanced is natural language processing, which can be considered as the ability of computers to understand text, including the subtle nuances it contains. Increasingly neural networking techniques are being used to allow computers to understand and even respond to written text.

Unsurprisingly, in the business arena those wishing to earn money have been quick to utilize such methods. For example, customer emails can be analysed to learn about customer desire and motivation (Coussement et al. 2008). Research into the analysis of texts in order to predict the movement of stocks and shares has also, inevitably, been conducted (Galvez et al. 2017).

HealthTweets.org

Developed by researchers based at John Hopkins Hospital Baltimore, HealthTweets.org is a platform presenting health related research from Twitter (Dredze et al. 2013). Data is streamed directly from Twitter, then using a statistical classifier those Tweets relating to health related matters are extracted. This system is based on 269 keywords, which are known from previous research to provide an indication of those Tweets containing health related stories. Using the Carmen geo-locating package, the location of these health related Tweets can be determined.

The data is then visualized in time series and map formats. It is possible to plot trends over time and compare levels of Tweeting in one location to another. Maps are also produced showing summaries of Tweets from different areas and thus allowing easy comparison.

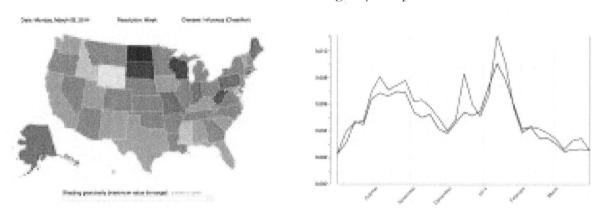

Taken from Dredze et al. (2013). The above figures show how HealthTweets.org provides the trend and geographical location of Tweets related to a specific condition. This helps those studying trends and patterns in disease occurrence.

News stories are infectious

In some respects news stories are themselves like an infectious disease; important news spreads from person to person, quickly transversing the globe. Early research concentrated on examining the first mention of news stories and how these later spread in popularity (Lerman and Ghosh, 2010). This is important in understanding the inter-relationship between media news coverage and actual disease occurrence.

RESEARCH EXAMPLES USING TWITTER

Here are some interesting examples where social media posts have been used to examine various health issues.

Chikungunya

Rocklöv et al. (2019) showed how using geo-located tweets they could assess mobility patterns in Italy. From this they assessed which areas were at greatest risk of chikungunya disease spreading from an outbreak centred around Rome and Anzio.

Measles and Ebola

Jahanbin et al. (2019) used both online news reports and Twitter messages to examine coverage on measles and Ebola virus. The authors developed an algorithm entitled a 'Fuzzy Algorithm for Extraction, Monitoring, and Classification of Infectious Diseases' (FAEMC-ID) to monitor Tweets. They monitored news output and were able to classify the geographical location of news report. They found these corresponded well with data obtained from the Center for Disease Control.

Eating disorders and fitness trackers

McCraig et al. (2018) is an example of the use of Twitter not related to disease. They studied online forums and examined the frequency fitness trackers were mentioned in eating disorder forums on the social media platform Reddit. Personal control over physical activity takes on an over proportional importance to those with eating disorders. They examined how often words related to fitness tracking were mentioned, finding that a pro-anorexia website mentioned them to a greater extent than those anorexia websites with a focus more on recovery. The identification of such trends helps understand such conditions better and identify sources of misinformation.

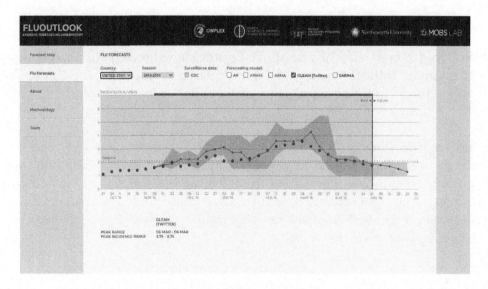

The website 'Fluoutlook' integrated data from Twitter to produce forecasts of influenza. Here forecasts for the U.S. using Twitter data.

Example studies using social media data to study disease outbreaks:

Study	Details
Allen et al. (2016)	Examined Tweeting rates about influenza for 30 U.S. cities and studied the relationship with official data. The study showed that there was a good correlation between Tweeting and actual number of influenza cases.
Gittelman et al. (2015)	Aggregated numbers of 'likes' in 37 facebook categories considered indicative of health for different U.S counties. They reduced these to nine important factors using Principal Component Analysis. Then they used regression analysis to show the factors fitted data on expected mortality as well as did socio-economic factors. A combined model using both Facebook and socio-economic factors had the best predictive value.
Harris et al. (2017)	The Healthmap dashboard was set to monitor Tweets on food borne illness around St. Louis. Tweets mentioning food poisoning related terms were classified by machine learning methods and by humans. Most food poisoning cases go unreported, and this increased identification of cases.
McGough et al. (2017)	Examined the 2015–2016 Latin American outbreak of Zika virus. They used a sample of Twitter posts and searched for mention of the words 'Zika', 'microcephaly', and 'microcefalia' with data being available for Colombia and Venezuela. Use of Twitter data in various models was examined and in some cases proved more effective than models without it.
Signorini et al. (2011)	Tracked public interest in H1N1 and influenza for the U.S. using Tweets. Used Tweet numbers to estimate both national and regional levels of influenza. These provided accurate forecasts two weeks before official data.

Advantages:
Some of the advantages that Twitter offers for the disease epidemiologist are:

- **Demographic and location data:** Tweets contain more information than other digital data sources such as results from Web searches. For example, Tweets can be geo-located providing useful indication of where they originate from. Additionally, it is easier to obtain demographic information about those sending Tweets than with other forms of digital surveillance.

- **Text information:** Despite being short, those posting messages about illness might provide useful additional information about the symptoms they experience. This means that filtering out of erroneous messages can occur. It also opens up the opportunity for different types of analysis. For example, keywords indicating the severity of illness could be studied, or potentially unknown symptoms could be identified.

- **Reaching the places normal epidemiology does not reach:** A big advantage of Twitter and other social media platforms is that they allow study of specific population groups, which often can't be reached with conventional methods (Alshaikh et al. 2014). Some groups may be reluctant to participate in health research, and even access healthcare provision at all, for a variety of social reasons (Silenzio et al. 2009). Use of social media potentially reaches such marginalized groups.

- **Speed:** People are likely to 'tweet' about how they feel even if they are only slightly ill or simply off. This means Tweets could offer an important first indication of an outbreak occurring. People only normally seek medical advice when they feel very poorly. Thus social media information could potentially pre-empt other forms of surveillance.

Disadvantages:
However, there are possible disadvantages:

- **Analysis investment:** Some other data sources, such as internet search results, are simple to access and analyse. In many cases such data is comprised of a single univariate time-series. Although the amount of information this contains is limited, it is at least easy to investigate and for researchers to work with. Content analysis of social media messages requires more complex techniques involving text mining and natural language processing. This requires some specialist knowledge and expertise.

- **News:** A number of studies have noted the problem that significant news events skew the content of messages. Obviously, when there is some major news event, it dominates social media messages, potentially drowning out the disease signals a scientist is seeking. Another issue is that when disease becomes news-worthy, such as when there is an anthrax bio-terrorism attack, a large number of social media posts relating to it will be sent with most coming from those not directly affected.

- **Self-selection bias:** Although social media messages might allow specific hard-to-reach groups to be targeted there comes the problem of self-selection bias. Not everyone has access to social media, not everyone chooses to post on it. What is different about those that do?

Where next?
HealthTweets.org showed how social media data could be used to produce a dashboard of use for those responsible for syndromic surveillance. The next research steps using Twitter and other social media sites is to determine those conditions where the incidence mirrors social media data, and to determine which keywords are most useful in ascertaining such trends. Once this has been done a true system of monitoring social media output can be developed.

REFERENCES

Allen C, Tsou MH, Aslam A, Nagel A, Gawron JM. Applying GIS and machine learning methods to Twitter data for multiscale surveillance of influenza. *Plos one*. 2016;**11**(7):e0157734.

Alshaikh F, Ramzan F, Rawaf S, Majeed A. Social network sites as a mode to collect health data: a systematic review. *Journal of medical internet research*. 2014;**16**(7):e171.

Aramaki E, Maskawa S, Morita M. Twitter catches the flu: detecting influenza epidemics using Twitter. In: Proceedings of the 2011 Conference on empirical methods in natural language processing 2011 Jul (pp. 1568-1576).

Chew C, Eysenbach G. Pandemics in the age of Twitter: content analysis of Tweets during the 2009 H1N1 outbreak. *Plos one*. 2010;**5**(11):e14118.

Coussement K, Van den Poel D. Integrating the voice of customers through call center emails into a decision support system for churn prediction. *Information management*. 2008;**45**(3):164-174.

Culotta A. Towards detecting influenza epidemics by analyzing Twitter messages. In: Proceedings of the first workshop on social media analytics 2010 Jul 25 (pp. 115-122).

Dredze M, Paul MJ, Bergsma S, Tran H. Carmen. A twitter geolocation system with applications to public health. In: Workshops at the twenty-seventh AAAI conference on artificial intelligence. 2013.

Gálvez RH, Gravano A. Assessing the usefulness of online message board mining in automatic stock prediction systems. *Journal of computing science*. 2017;**19**:43–56.

Gittelman S, Lange V, Crawford CA, Okoro CA, Lieb E, Dhingra SS, Trimarchi E. A new source of data for public health surveillance: Facebook likes. *Journal of medical internet research*. 2015;**17**(4):e3970.

Harris JK, Hawkins JB, Nguyen L, Nsoesie EO, Tuli G, Mansour R, Brownstein JS. Research brief report: Using twitter to identify and respond to food poisoning: The food safety stl project. *Journal of public health management and practice*. 2017;**23**(6):577.

Jahanbin K, Rahmanian F, Rahmanian V, Jahromi AS. Application of Twitter and web news mining in infectious disease surveillance systems and prospects for public health. *GMS hygiene and infection control*. 2019;**14**.

Lerman K, Ghosh R. Information contagion: An empirical study of the spread of news on digg and twitter social networks. In: Fourth international AAAI conference on weblogs and social media 2010 May 16.

McCaig D, Bhatia S, Elliott MT, Walasek L, Meyer C. Text-mining as a methodology to assess eating disorder-relevant factors: Comparing mentions of fitness tracking technology across online communities. *International journal of eating disorders*. 2018;**51**(7):647-55.

McGough SF, Brownstein JS, Hawkins JB, Santillana M. Forecasting Zika incidence in the 2016 Latin America outbreak combining traditional disease surveillance with search, social media, and news report data. *Plos neglected tropical diseases*. 2017;**11**(1):e0005295.

Paul MJ, Dredze M. You are what you tweet: Analyzing twitter for public health. In: Fifth International AAAI Conference on Weblogs and Social Media 2011.

Post A. How many social media posts are published each day. 2022. Available at: www.socialmediadata.com/how-many-social-media-posts-are-published-each-day/

Rocklöv J, Tozan Y, Ramadona A, Sewe MO, Sudre B, Garrido J, de Saint Lary CB, Lohr W, Semenza JC. Using big data to monitor the introduction and spread of Chikungunya, Europe, 2017. *Emerging infectious diseases*. 2019;**25**(6):1041.

Signorini A, Segre AM, Polgreen PM. The use of Twitter to track levels of disease activity and public concern in the U.S. during the influenza A H1N1 pandemic. *Plos one.* 2011;**6**(5): e19467.

Silenzio VM, Duberstein PR, Tang W, Lu N, Tu X, Homan CM. Connecting the invisible dots: reaching lesbian, gay, and bisexual adolescents and young adults at risk for suicide through online social networks. *Social science and medicine.* 2009;**69**(3):469-474.

15

WIKIPEDIA

Imagine a world in which every single person on the planet
is given free access to the sum of all human knowledge

Jimmy Wales, founder of Wikipedia.

Wikipedia is an online encyclopedia with a twist. Anyone can be a writer or editor. Text can be written or corrected by those actually using the encyclopedia. The idea is that with the input from enough people, that through a process of iteration articles will be gradually improved and kept updated. Mistakes will be ironed out. A democratic encyclopedia!

Launched in 2001 by Jimmy Wales and Larry Sanger, Wikipedia aimed to give the power of knowledge to people. Traditionally, encyclopedias are written by 'experts'. These decide what to include and how to present it. But who is an 'expert'? And who decides who is an 'expert' and who is not? Does that mean the ideas and knowledge of 'non-experts' are not valid?

Another important consideration is the style of writing and tone used in texts. Often the manner in which something is presented can greatly influence how it is judged. Just think of how different media outlets, with different political agendas, present the same news stories to emphasize the points that best suit their own opinions. Traditionally, those employed to present news and information all came from similar backgrounds, all received educations from the same institutions, and thus all tended to have similar viewpoints. Wikipedia tried to dispense with this. It showed that anyone can play an active part in knowledge creation and dissemination, whoever they are, and wherever they come from. This means that different viewpoints get emphasized.

Studies have shown that Wikipedia is as accurate as traditional paper based encyclopedias (Giles, 2005). An additional advantage over paper based encyclopedias is the sheer size of Wikipedia. A paper based encyclopedia might contain a few hundred pages, maybe a few thousand at most. But the internet allows tens of thousands, if not potentially millions of articles to be created. This means knowledge is democratized in a different manner; people can choose themselves which pages to visit, instead of only being limited to those that editors believe are worthy enough to be included, as is the case with paper based published texts. In March 2022, there were 1.9 billion readers, 380,000 acted as editors and there were over 60 million page edits (Wikipedia Statistics, 2023). Another advantage is the ease of accessibility; it is possible to call up a Wikipedia page anywhere there is internet access. No need for a visit to the library. Information is there instantly.

Wikipedia does not offer the same scope for the disease biologist as other digital epidemiology data sources because the range of information collected about users is more limited. This is despite it becoming a widely used reference source for those seeking medical information; nearly 5 billion page views even in 2013 (Heilman and West, 2015). However, it has still been used in various ways to study various topics related to health and disease. The majority of scientific studies examining health related issues have studied the accuracy of the information on Wiki pages for various conditions (e.g. Kupferberg and Protus, 2011).

Page access views and influenza

McIver and Brownstein (2014) looked at whether the number of views a Wikipedia pages received was related to official influenza case numbers. Could this be used to make forecasts of the likely future number of influenza cases? They gathered the daily number of views made to pages on influenza related subjects, such as on the common cold. They then used a Poisson model with LASSO regression to fit the data and make forecasts.

Hickmann et al. (2015) also used weekly Wikipedia page views. They examined data from 50 pages, and found the best correlation between weekly official data on influenza-like-illness and page views was for data from the pages on 'human flu', 'influenza', 'influenza A virus' and 'influenza B virus'. They then integrated this data into linear models for influenza and were able to make credible predictions for the 2013-2014 influenza season.

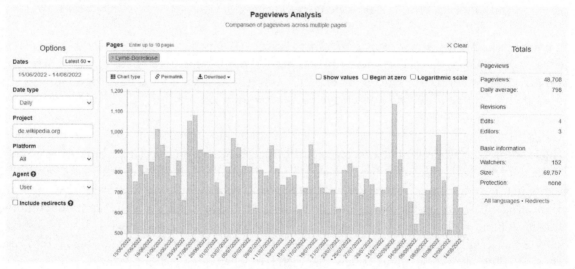

This figure shows the number of Wikipedia page views for the German page 'Lyme-borreliose' (lyme disease) over a 60 day period running from 15/06/2022. Interesting is that page views peak on Mondays. Lyme disease is a tick borne infection. Most people probably engage in outdoors activities over the weekends, and this is thus when they get bitten by ticks. It appears they search for information on Lyme disease shortly afterwards. The classic diagnostic feature of Lyme disease is a circular 'bulls eye' rash, which is most distinctive. However, although this can develop two days following a tick bite, it most typically develops about five days following such a bite. Thus it could be that people are searching for information out of fear infection and before the classic diagnostic symptom appears. This example illustrates how Wikipedia can be used to study aspects related to disease other data does not allow.

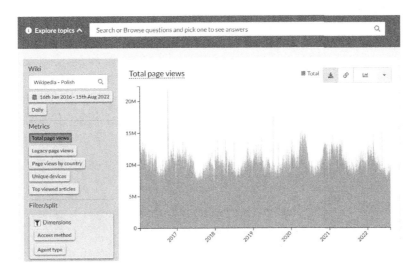

Above information from the 'statistics' of the Polish 'influenza' Wikipedia page. It shows a clear seasonal trend in page views corresponding to when influenza peaks.

Modelling with Wikipedia

Generous et al. (2014) modelled disease incidence for a number of infectious conditions using the page access logs which show the number of views pages received. The authors examined 14 different disease and location combinations. As geographical information on readers is not provided from this information, they used language as a proxy for location. A number of languages are limited in the area in which they are used allowing this to be inferred. For example, the Thai language is predominately used only in the country of Thailand. They selected top articles related to each condition, then used linear modelling to produce forecasts for the expected disease incidence.

The results proved to be context specific. Models using Wikipedia views were successful at forecasting conditions such as dengue fever in Thailand, influenza in Japan, influenza in Thailand, and tuberculosis in Thailand. However, other models were less effective, such as for HIV/AIDS in Japan and tuberculosis in Norway. This emphasizes the need to refine models for each context.

Advantages and disadvantages

An advantage of Wikipedia data is that page access views can be obtained for the daily time scale, which can be most useful when wanting to determine the current picture and be as up-to-date as possible. It also allows trends that might vary on a daily basis, such as over the weekend, to be studied. The main disadvantage of Wikipedia data is that the amount of information that Wikipedia provides is somewhat limited; it is not possible to obtain data on where page views are occurring and the type of user doing such viewing. This limits the type of analysis that is possible using Wikipedia.

REFERENCES

Generous N, Fairchild G, Deshpande A, Del Valle SY, Priedhorsky R. Global disease monitoring and forecasting with Wikipedia. *Plos computational biology.* 2014;**10**(11):e1003892.

Giles J. Internet encyclopaedias go head to head. *Nature.* 2005;**438**:900-901.

Heilman JM, West AG. Wikipedia and medicine: quantifying readership, editors, and the significance of natural language. *Journal of medical internet research.* 2015;**17**(3):e4069.

Hickmann KS, Fairchild G, Priedhorsky R, Generous N, Hyman JM, Deshpande A, Del Valle SY. Forecasting the 2013–2014 influenza season using Wikipedia. *Plos computational biology.* 2015;**11**(5):e1004239.

McIver D, Brownstein J. Wikipedia usage estimates prevalence of influenza-like illness in the United States in near real-time. *Plos computational biology.* 2014;**10**:1-8.

Kupferberg N, Protus BM. Accuracy and completeness of drug information in Wikipedia: An assessment. *Journal of the medical library association.* 2011; **99**:310-313.

Wikipedia. Statistics. 2023. Available at: https://stats.wikimedia.org/#/en.wikipedia.org

THE COVID REVOLUTION

We have it totally under control. It's one person coming in from China.
It's going to be just fine.

Donald Trump on COVID-19,
January 2020.

The COVID-19 viral infection was identified in late 2019 and spread around the world in 2020. The condition is officially entitled coronavirus disease 2019, but is usually commonly named as COVID-19. It signalled an important milestone in the development of digital epidemiology. Disease outbreaks and pandemics of importance had been occurring regularly during the previous two decades. For example, the H1N1 'swine flu' influenza pandemic swept the globe in 2009, and an outbreak of Severe Acute Respiratory Syndrome (SARS) occurred between 2002 and 2004. However, COVID-19 was different because of the truly global nature of the pandemic, its perceived severity, and the profound economic and social impact it is having globally. It can also be argued that this is the first digital pandemic. The widespread availability of internet connectivity and other digital resources meant this was the first pandemic which could be tracked, monitored and studied globally.

By December 2020 the official death toll stood at 1,813,188 (WHO, 2022). Many people cite warfare as being an accelerator of human progress and ingenuity. Maybe the same can be said of pandemics in the epidemiological research sphere? Research efforts globally were directed towards understanding, tracking and monitoring this disease. Many of the methods of studying the spread of COVID-19 used technologies mentioned previously in this book.

What were the important digital epidemiological resources that were developed throughout the pandemic? Here are a selection, which are meant to provide an idea. As time passes it will be easier to evaluate the different advances that occurred during this period better.

Contact tracing

One of the notable developments during the COVID-19 pandemic was the use and development of contact tracing (O'Neill et al. 2020). Traditionally, contract tracing is what epidemiologists do in order to trace the origins of an outbreak and ascertain all the people who might be infected. It involves a lot of questioning and traditionally a lot of feet-on-the-ground epidemiology.

Obviously new technology offers a chance to automate the process. Although in development prior to the COVID-19 pandemic, interest in specialised apps facilitating contact tracing exploded in 2020. Ahmed et al. (2020) provides an introduction to contract tracing, detailing how it is performed and how such apps can be developed. There was some evidence to suggest such contact tracing could reduce transmission (Ferretti et al. 2020).

Most contact tracing apps utilise Bluetooth technology for proximity estimation between devices. Ahmed et al. (2020) describes three main forms; centralised, decentralised and a hybrid approach. In the centralised approach a user registers and downloads an app, which provides a temporary ID which is encrypted using a secret key. When mobile devices come into close contact with each other these temporary ID's are exchanged between them. Each device records encounters and stores them locally. Should a user test positive for COVID-19 then records can be uploaded to the central server, and all contacts to that device be informed.

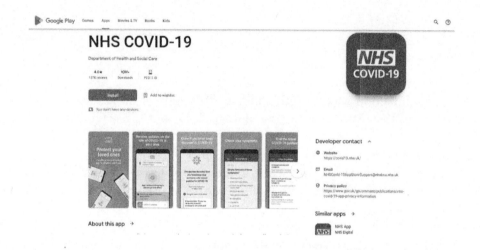

The NHS COVID app available for download on Google Play. U.K. Health Security Agency (2023).

John Hopkins COVID-19 dashboard

The data resources collated by the John Hopkins University (JHU, 2023) were quickly recognized worldwide as providing a gold standard which could be used to assess the impact the disease was having globally. The initial dashboard provided data on the number of confirmed cases and deaths attributed to the condition (Dong et al. 2020). For researchers wanting an overview, this resource became one of the most heavily used and cited.

Right: The John Hopkins COVID-19 dashboard.

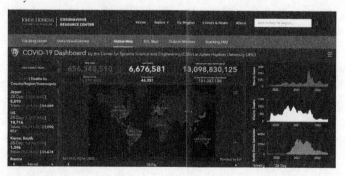

The CDC COVID-19 data tracker

Also extensive in the amount of data it provided is the Center for Disease Control (CDC) COVID-19 data tracker, which although U.S. based, provides wide range of data including on specific ethnic and gender groups affected by COVID-19 (CDC, 2023).

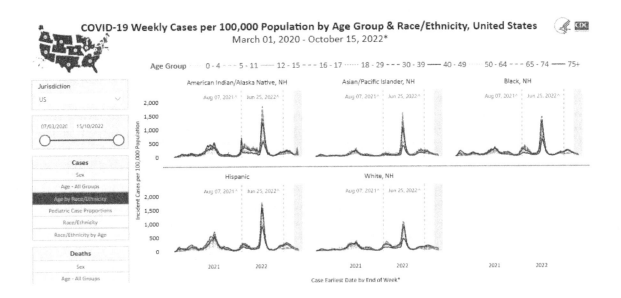

Syndromic surveillance of COVID-19

Launched in the U.K. on the 24th of March and in the U. S. on the 29th March 2020, the COVID-19 Symptom Tracker was a syndromic surveillance system for COVID-19 symptoms (Drew et al. 2020). Through use of this app users self report symptoms. Initially it asks users to provide their location and such basic information as their age. 1,6 million participants were using this in the first five days of its implementation.

From March 2020 the data this system provided proved invaluable in identifying geographical locations where symptoms were most prevalent. It quickly showed that the most common symptoms were fatigue and a cough. It also showed areas of the U.K. where complex symptoms were most common and where positive tests were concentrated. When one considers that a major concern at this time was that the health system could be overwhelmed, such information was important in understanding where problems might develop first and how resource allocation could be managed.

Typically, symptoms develop before testing occurs and cases are confirmed. Predictive modelling using reported symptoms was able to predict when peaks in confirmed cases would occur. For example, in southern Wales rises in reported symptoms occurred between five and seven days prior to corresponding peaks in confirmed cases.

Government restrictions

Hale et al. (2020) produced a dataset detailing the level of restrictions on different aspects of life across the globe. This dataset allowed the severity of restrictions to be compared between countries. It also allowed study of whether the severity of restrictions was related to transmission of the virus.

Studying mobility and COVID-19

The potential of using technology to study the links between mobility and COVID-19 was identified early in the pandemic (Buckee et al. 2020; Oliver et al. 2020). One of the earliest studies to do so was Kraemer et al. (2020). This study used data from the Chinese technology company Baidu on the volume of travel leaving Wuhan to model the course the epidemic would take. This study found that the amount of travel away from Wuhan influenced the magnitude of the epidemic. The size of epidemics in neighbouring areas depended on the amount of travel from Wuhan which seeded them. This study thus showed the importance of travel restrictions in combating the spread of COVID-19.

As detailed in the chapter on smartphone surveillance, access to data is a major constraint limiting study of the link between mobility and disease. In order to facilitate study of how mobility influences COVID-19 transmission, large technology companies were ready to share the data they had. Google released data through its Community Mobility Reports, which detailed levels of society mobility at key location categories both at national and regional levels (Google, 2020). Apple's Mobility Reports (Apple, 2020) showed mobility levels by providing data on those making direction requests when either driving, in transit, or walking. These datasets used information sourced from personal mobile phone records in an anonymised format. Digital epidemiologists were quick to utilise these resources to show how mobility and COVID-19 were related.

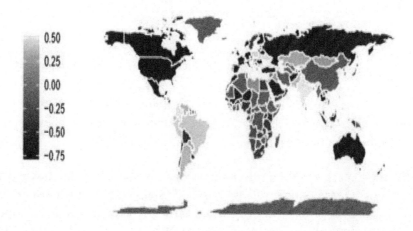

Resources such as the Google Community Mobility Reports allowed the relationship between community mobility and COVID-19 case numbers to be investigated. Here the correlation between 'transit' hub activity in Google's Community Mobility Reports and official COVID-19 cases from October 2020. Adapted from: Sulyok and Walker (2020).

Excess deaths

Official figures as to the number of deaths from COVID-19 underestimate the true total. In some countries cases go undiagnosed due to lack of resources. In others there may be political reasons why authorities wish to downplay the importance of COVID-19. Even in countries where one might think good records might be kept, there could be reasons why reported figures do not truly reflect the actual number of deaths. For example, even in the U.K. there could be reluctance to list COVID-19 as the main cause of death. Deaths could occur not directly through COVID-19, but due to knock-on consequences of the pandemic, for example problems in accessing the healthcare system due to 'lockdowns', or due to reduced capacity which could result in increases in deaths from other reasons.

A way to estimate the true picture is to examine excess deaths and how these compare to other periods in time. A noted resource for study of excess deaths during COVID-19 is the Economist Excess death tracker. This simply examines the number of deaths in excess of the baseline levels. In the case of the Economist they used a five year moving average to ascertain the baseline.

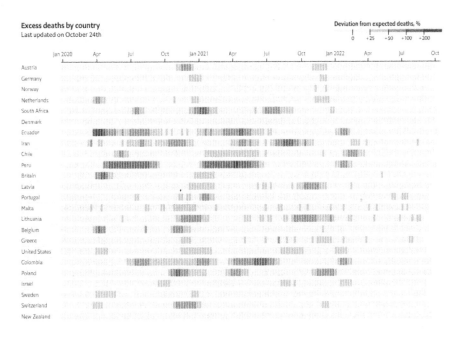

**The Economist Excess Death
Tracker (Economist, 2023).**

Where next?

The COVID-19 pandemic maybe emphasised how much there still is to do digitally. The disparity in officially reported deaths and the number estimated to have died shows how much improvement is needed in the recording and monitoring of disease. WHO estimated that excess deaths in 2020 resulting from COVID-19 were over three million. This compared to the official figure for deaths from COVID-19 of 1.8 million (WHO, 2022). Although 98% of deaths were recorded in

European countries, in African countries only 10% were recorded officially. It is likely that the number of cases reported from Africa was severely below what actually occurred.

COVID-19 also emphasised that epidemiologists have a greater role than simply collecting and interpreting data. An additional and very important role is in providing information, and arguably fighting misinformation. Unorthodox ideas regarding the virus and vaccination were widely propagated. During the early stages of the pandemic social media was important in informing the public about COVID-19 and combatting the false ideas that were circulating (Zarcostas, 2020).

Another pandemic will occur and spread to affect a large number of people globally. This is inevitable. Were we prepared for COVID-19? The varied and panicked responses by governments globally indicated that we were not. However, the speed at which many of the research programs outlined in this chapter were implemented, shows that the knowledge and background infrastructure required were already in place.

To read official health reports one might believe that disease surveillance still occurs only through official channels, with outbreaks being 'picked up' by healthcare professionals in professional healthcare settings. But this is no longer the case. WHO now recognises that informal sources of information are as important as official ones. In fact more so. The WHO Alert and Response operations unit recently stated that more than 60% of the first reports of an disease outbreak come from informal and often unofficial sources (WHO, 2020). Will we be better prepared for the next pandemic? COVID-19 shows that development of these informal information sources is vital so that we are better placed to combat the next pandemic that will occur.

When we work with numbers on a screen, downloaded from a website, it is easy to forget why we are doing this and what the numbers mean. We can't be perfect, we will make mistakes, but it is important to act with honesty and do the best we can. I want to finish with the following statement, which acts as motivation to act with integrity, and a reminder and motivation for why we are doing what we do:

We must remember that behind every health figure is a person, a family – a life. Data on loss of life is no different.

WHO, The True Death Toll From COVID-19

REFERENCES
Ahmed N, Michelin RA, Xue W, Ruj S, Malaney R, Kanhere SS, Seneviratne A, Hu W, Janicke H, Jha SK. A survey of COVID-19 contact tracing apps. *IEEE access.* 2020;8:134577-601.

Apple. Mobility trend reports. 2020. Available at: https://covid19.apple.com/ mobility

Buckee CO, Balsari S, Chan J, Crosas M, Dominici F, Gasser U, Grad YH, Grenfell B, Halloran ME, Kraemer MU, Lipsitch M. Aggregated mobility data could help fight COVID-19. *Science.* 2020;368:145-146.

Center for Disease Control (CDC). COVID Data Tracker. 2023. Available at: https://covid.cdc.gov/covid-data-tracker/

Dong E, Du H, Gardner L. An interactive web-based dashboard to track COVID-19 in real time. The l*ancet infectious diseases*. 2020;20:533-534.

Drew DA, Nguyen LH, Steves CJ, Menni C, Freydin M, Varsavsky T, Sudre CH, Cardoso MJ, Ourselin S, Wolf J, Spector TD. Rapid implementation of mobile technology for real-time epidemiology of COVID-19. *Science*. 2020;**368**:1362-1367

Economist. Excess Death Tracker. 2023. Available at: www.economist.com/graphic-detail/coronavirus-excess-deaths-tracker

Ferretti L, Wymant C, Kendall M, Zhao L, Nurtay A, Abeler-Dörner L, Parker M, Bonsall D, Fraser C. Quantifying SARS-CoV-2 transmission suggests epidemic control with digital contact tracing. *Science*. 2020;**368**(6491).

Google. Google community mobility reports. 2020. Available at: www.google.com/covid19/mobility/

Hale T, Angrist N, Kira B, Petherick A, Phillips T, Webster S. Variation in government responses to COVID-19. Blavatnik school of government working paper, 31. 2020. Available at https:// www.bsg.ox.ac.uk/research/publications/variation-government-responsescovid-19

John Hopkins University (JHU). Coronavirus Resource Center. 2023
Available at: https://coronavirus.jhu.edu/map.html

Kraemer MU, Yang CH, Gutierrez B, Wu CH, Klein B, Pigott DM, Open COVID-19 Data Working Group, Du Plessis L, Faria NR, Li R, Hanage WP. The effect of human mobility and control measures on the COVID-19 epidemic in China. *Science*. 2020;**368**(6490):493-7.

Oliver N, Letouzé E, Sterly H, Delataille S, De Nadai M, Lepri B, Lambiotte R, Benjamins R, Cattuto C, Colizza V, de Cordes N. Mobile phone data and COVID-19: missing an opportunity? *ArXiv*. 2020;2003.12347.

O'Neill PH, Ryan-Mosley T, Johnson B. A flood of coronavirus apps are tracking us. Now it's time to keep track of them. *MIT technology review*. 2020. Available at: www.technologyreview.com/2020/05/07/1000961/launching-mit-tr-covid-tracing-tracker/

Sulyok M, Walker M. Community movement and COVID-19: a global study using Google's community mobility reports. *Epidemiology and infection*. 2020;**148**.

World Health Organization (WHO). Epidemic intelligence - systematic event detection. 2020. Available at: https://www.who.int/csr/alertresponse/epidemicintelligence/en/

World Health Organization (WHO). The true death toll of COVID-19. Estimating global excess mortality. 2022. Available at: www.who.int/data/stories/the-true-death-toll-of-covid-19-estimating-global-excess-mortality

U.K. Health Security Agency. The NHS COVID app. 2023. Available at: www.gov.uk/government/collections/nhs-covid-19-app

Zarcostos J. How to fight an infodemic. *The lancet*. 2020;**395**(10225):676.